Praise for
THE
and

"The concept of the glycemic index has been distorted and bastardized by popular writers and diet gurus. Here, at last, is a book that explains what we know about the glycemic index and its importance in designing a diet for optimum health. Carbohydrates are not all bad. Read the good news about pasta and even—believe it or not—sugar!"

—ANDREW WEIL, M.D., University of Arizona College of Medicine,
author of *Spontaneous Healing* and *8 Weeks to Optimum Health*,
on *The Glucose Revolution*

■

"Forget *SugarBusters*. Forget *The Zone*. If you want the real scoop on how carbohydrates and sugar affect your body, read this book by the world's leading researchers on the subject. It's the authoritative, last word on choosing foods to control your blood sugar."

—JEAN CARPER, best-selling author of
Miracle Cures, Stop Aging Now!, and *Food: Your Miracle Medicine*,
on *The Glucose Revolution*

■

"Clear, accessible, and authoritative information about the glycemic index. An exciting, new approach to preventing obesity, diabetes, and heart disease—written by internationally recognized experts in the field."

—DAVID LUDWIG, M.D., PH.D., director, Obesity Program,
Children's Hospital, Boston, on *The New Glucose Revolution*

■

"Mounting evidence indicates that refined carbohydrates and high glycemic index foods are contributing to the escalating epidemics of obesity and type 2 diabetes worldwide. This dietary pattern also appears to increase the risk of heart disease and stroke. The skyrocketing proportion of calories from added sugars and refined carbohydrates in Westernized diets portends a future acceleration of these trends. *The Glucose Revolution* challenges traditional doctrines about optimal nutrition and the role of carbohydrates in health and disease. Brand-Miller and colleagues are to be congratulated for an eminently lucid and important book that explains the science behind the glycemic index and provides tools and strategies for modifying diet to incorporate this knowledge. I strongly recommend the book to both health professionals and the general public who could use this state-of-the-art information to improve health and well-being."

—JOANN E. MANSON, M.D., DR.P.H., professor of medicine,
Harvard Medical School and codirector of Women's Health,
Division of Preventive Medicine, Brigham and Women's Hospital

■

"Here is at last a book explaining the importance of taking into consideration the glycemic index values of foods for overall health, athletic performance, and in reducing the risk of heart disease and diabetes. The book clearly explains that there are different kinds of carbohydrates that work in different ways and why a universal recommendation to 'increase the carbohydrate content of your diet' is plainly simple and scientifically inaccurate. Everyone should put the glycemic index approach into practice."

—ARTEMIS P. SIMOPOULOS, M.D., senior author of
The Omega Diet and *The Healing Diet* and president,
The Center for Genetics, Nutrition and Health,
Washington, D.C., on *The Glucose Revolution*

■

"*The Glucose Revolution* is nutrition science for the twenty-first century. Clearly written, it gives the scientific rationale for why all carbohydrates are not created equal. It is a practical guide for both professionals and patients. The food suggestions and recipes are exciting and tasty."

—RICHARD N. PODELL, M.D., M.P.H., clinical professor,
Department of Family Medicine, UMDNJ-Robert Wood Johnson
Medical School, and coauthor of *The G-Index Diet: The Missing Link
That Makes Permanent Weight Loss Possible*

"The glycemic index is a useful tool which may have a broad spectrum of applications, from the maintenance of fuel supply during exercise to the control of blood glucose levels in diabetics. Low glycemic index foods may prove to have beneficial health effects for all of us in the long term. *The Glucose Revolution* is a user-friendly, easy-to-read overview of all that you need to know about the glycemic index. This book represents a balanced account of the importance of the glycemic index based on sound scientific evidence."

—JAMES HILL, PH.D., director, Center for Human Nutrition, University of Colorado Health Sciences Center

∎

"*The New Glucose Revolution* summarizes much of the recent development of dietary glycemic index and load in a highly readable format. The authors are able researchers and respected leaders in the nutrition field. Much that is discussed in this book draws directly from their years of experimental and observational research. The focus on dietary intervention and prevention strategies in everyday eating is an especially laudable feature of this book. I recommend this book most highly as an indispensable source of good nutrition."

—SIMIN LIU, M.D., SC.D., assistant professor, Department of Epidemiology, Harvard School of Public Health

∎

"As a coach of elite amateur and professional athletes, I know how critical the glycemic index is to sports performance. *The New Glucose Revolution* provides the serious athlete with the basic tools necessary for getting the training table right."

—JOE FRIEL, coach, author, consultant

Other Glucose Revolution & New Glucose Revolution Titles

The New Glucose Revolution: The Authoritative Guide to the Glycemic Index—The Dietary Solution for Lifelong Health

The Glucose Revolution Life Plan

What Makes My Blood Glucose Go Up . . . And Down? And 101 Other Frequently Asked Questions about Your Blood Glucose Levels

The New Glucose Revolution Complete Guide to Glycemic Index Values

The New Glucose Revolution Pocket Guide to the Top 100 Low GI Foods

The New Glucose Revolution Pocket Guide to Diabetes

The New Glucose Revolution Pocket Guide to Losing Weight

The New Glucose Revolution Pocket Guide to the Metabolic Syndrome and Your Heart

The New Glucose Revolution Pocket Guide to Peak Performance

The New Glucose Revolution Poceket Guide to Healthy Kids

■

The Glucose Revolution Pocket Guide to Sugar and Energy

■

FORTHCOMING

The New Glucose Revolution Life Plan

The New Glucose Revolution Smart Carb Diet

The New Glucose Revolution Guide to Managing PCOS

The New Glucose Revolution Pocket Guide to Sugar and Energy

The NEW GLUCOSE Revolution

POCKET GUIDE TO CHILDHOOD DIABETES

Jennie Brand-Miller, Ph.D.
Kaye Foster-Powell, M. Nutr. & Diet.
Heather Gilbertson, B. Sc., Grad. Dip. Diet., Grad. Cert. Ed., APD

Marlowe & Company
New York

THE NEW GLUCOSE REVOLUTION POCKET GUIDE TO CHILDHOOD DIABETES

Copyright © 1997, 2004 by Jennie Brand-Miller,
Kaye Foster-Powell, Heather Gilbertson

Published by
Marlowe & Company
An Imprint of Avalon Publishing Group Incorporated
245 West 17th Street • 11th Floor
New York, NY 10011-5300

This edition was published in somewhat different form in Australia in 2003 under the title *The New Glucose Revolution Childhood Diabetes* by Hodder Headline Australia Pty Limited. This edition is published by arrangement with Hodder Headline Australia Pty Limited.

The GI logo is a trademark of the University of Sydney in Australia and other countries. A food product carrying this logo is nutritious and has been tested for its GI by an accredited laboratory.

All rights reserved. No part of this book may be reproduced in whole or in part without written permission from the publisher, except by reviewers who may quote brief excerpts in connection with a review in a newspaper, magazine, or electronic publication; nor may any part of this book be reproduced, stored in a retrieval system, or transmitted in any form or by any means electronic, mechanical, photocopying, recording, or other, without written permission from the publisher.

ISBN 1-56924-430-8

9 8 7 6 5 4 3 2 1

Designed by Pauline Neuwirth, Neuwirth & Associates, Inc.
Printed in the United States of America
Distributed by Publishers Group West

CONTENTS

Preface	xi
How to Use This Book	xiii

PART 1:
The Glucose Revolution and Diabetes

1	What is the Glucose Revolution?	3
2	The Glycemic Index and Diabetes	5
3	Diabetes and Carbohydrates	8
4	What Type of Carbohydrate?	11
5	Sources of Carbohydrate	13
6	Why We Need More Carbohydrate	14
7	The Glycemic Index: Some Background	16
8	How We Measure the Glycemic Index	20

PART 2: The Glycemic Index and Your Child

9. Low-GI Diets for Children — 25
10. Who Benefits from Low-GI Foods? — 27
11. The Food Pyramid for Children — 29
12. Blood Sugar and Exercise — 31
13. Blood-Sugar Guidelines — 34
14. Handling Low Blood Sugar — 36
15. Sick Day Hypoglycemia — 40

PART 3: Food Basics

16. Cereals and Grain Foods — 47
17. Vegetables — 51
18. Fruit — 52
19. Dairy Foods — 54
20. Meat and Meat Alternatives — 56
21. Fats and Oils — 58
22. Sugar — 60

PART 4: Age-Specific Information for Diabetic Children

23. Babies — 67
24. Toddlers and Pre-Schoolers — 72
25. School-Age Children — 76
26. Teenagers — 80

POCKET GUIDE TO CHILDHOOD DIABETES

| 27 | **The Food Pyramid for Adolescents and Teenagers** | 88 |

PART 5:
The Glycemic Index Menu Planner for Children and Teens

28	**Breakfast**	93
29	**Lunches and Sandwich Fillers**	96
30	**Main Meals for Children and Teens**	99
31	**Just Desserts**	103
32	**Low-GI Snacks**	105
33	**Party Ideas**	107
34	**Other Low-GI Diets**	109

PART 6:
Your Questions Answered

35	**The Meal Skippers**	115
	No Special Treats Required	117
	Candy Concerns	118
	Hypoglycemia After Sports	118
	Infant and Toddler Concerns	119

PART 7:
The GI Tables

36	**Let's Talk Glycemic Load**	125
37	**A to Z GI Values**	129
38	**Your Low-GI Food Finder**	147
39	**Low- to High-GI Values**	152

THE NEW GLUCOSE REVOLUTION

For More Information — 170
Glycemic Index Testing — 172
About the Authors — 173
Acknowledgments — 175

PREFACE

THE NEW GLUCOSE REVOLUTION and *The Glucose Revolution Life Plan* are the definitive, all-in-one guides to the glycemic index. To supplement that information, we've now written this pocket guide to show you how the glycemic index relates to children with either type 1 or type 2 diabetes. We'll describe how the glycemic index can reduce blood-sugar levels and show you how easy it is to choose low-GI foods that benefit your whole family.

About one in every 400 to 500 children has type 1 diabetes. And although type 2 diabetes used to be considered rare among children, research indicates that this illness is becoming more common among children and adolescents, particularly in American Indians, African Americans, and Hispanics / Latinos.

In this volume, we offer more in-depth information about how the glycemic index affects children with diabetes than we had room to include in our other books: For example, we've included the questions that people most frequently ask about children's diabetes, nutrition, and many other extras. For a more comprehensive discussion of the glycemic index and all its uses, please consult *The New Glucose Revolution* and *The Glucose Revolution Life Plan*.

Please note: We have used the pronoun "she" throughout this book when describing a child with diabetes. We chose to use this word only in the interest of consistency, not to exclude boys or to imply in any way that girls are the only children affected by the disease.

HOW TO USE THIS BOOK

MANY YOUNG PEOPLE with diabetes, despite doing everything they are told, often find that their blood-sugar levels remain too high. This pocket guide will help you to understand the glycemic index and how you can use it to help your child with diabetes. After eating the low-GI way, your children will be well on the road to a lifetime of healthy eating that will help them to control their blood sugar and avoid diabetic complications. In this book, we:

- explain which types of carbohydrate are best for children with diabetes and why;
- show you how to include more of the right sort of carbohydrate in your child's diet;
- provide practical hints for meal preparation and tips to help make the glycemic index work throughout the day;

- give you lots of low-GI menus that children (even picky eaters) will love; and
- include an A to Z listing of over 300 foods with their GI values, carbohydrate, and fat grams.

■

This book contains the latest information about carbohydrates and the optimum diet for children with diabetes.

■

PART 1

THE GLUCOSE REVOLUTION AND DIABETES

1

WHAT IS THE GLUCOSE REVOLUTION?

*I*N OUR BOOK, *The New Glucose Revolution*, we explained that not all carbohydrates are created equal, and discussed how different types of carbohydrate work in different ways in our bodies. We revealed that some carbohydrates are absorbed much more slowly than others and that these slowly digested carbohydrates have startling health benefits for everybody. These carbohydrates:

- provide sustained energy;
- satisfy and reduce appetite;
- lower insulin levels, which makes you burn more—and store less—fat;
- help manage diabetes; and
- reduce diabetes, heart disease and certain cancer risks.

We also explained that eating the right *amount* of carbohydrate, as well as the right *type* of carbohydrate significantly contribute to our quality of life, health, and well-being.

The rate of carbohydrate digestion has important implications for everybody, but in this book we show how it can help young people with diabetes.

So whether you have diabetes yourself or care for someone who does, we believe that the GI value of carbohydrate foods is vital information that will help you with your day-to-day efforts at blood-sugar control.

Our research has been described as a "glucose revolution" because it has turned many traditional beliefs about starchy foods upside down and has changed the way we think about carbohydrates forever!

■

The glucose revolution can give young people with diabetes a new lease on life!

■

2

THE GLYCEMIC INDEX AND DIABETES

*N*OT LONG AGO, people with diabetes were told to eat complex carbohydrates (starches) because it was believed these were slowly absorbed, causing a smaller rise in blood-sugar levels. Doctors asked people with diabetes to restrict the amount of simple sugars they ate because these simple sugars were thought to be quickly absorbed, making blood sugar shoot up fast and high.

We now know that these assumptions were wrong. Different carbohydrate foods *do* have different effects on blood-sugar levels, but we can't predict the effect by looking at the sugar or starch content. We know this because since the 1980s scientists have studied the actual blood-sugar responses—of healthy people and people with diabetes—to hundreds of foods. Researchers asked people to eat everyday foods, then measured their blood-sugar levels frequently for two or three hours after the meal.

To rank carbohydrates according to their true physiological effect on blood-sugar levels, the scientists came up with the term "glycemic index." This is simply a ranking of foods from 0 to 100 that tells us whether a food will raise blood-sugar levels dramatically, moderately, or just a little.

The first surprise was that many starchy foods (bread, potatoes, crackers, and many breakfast cereals) are digested and absorbed very quickly, not slowly as we had once assumed.

The next surprise was that moderate amounts of many sugary foods did not produce dramatic rises in blood sugar that we had thought. In fact, many foods containing sugar actually showed intermediate blood-sugar responses, often lower than foods such as bread.

The glycemic index tells the true story: The old distinctions between starchy foods and sugary foods or simple versus complex carbohydrate have no scientific basis at all.

■

Forget about simple and complex carbohydrate, or good or bad foods. Think glucose revolution!

■

WHY IS THE GLYCEMIC INDEX SO IMPORTANT IN DIABETES?

When a person has diabetes and her blood sugar isn't under control, it can cause damage to the blood vessels in the heart, legs, brain, eyes, and kidneys. This is why heart attacks, strokes, kidney failure, and blindness are more common in people with diabetes. High blood-sugar levels can also damage the nerves in the feet, causing pain, irritation, and numbness.

Low-GI foods can help reduce the complications of diabetes by:

- improving blood-sugar control, and
- improving blood fats.

Several studies show that a low-GI diet lowers "bad" (LDL) cholesterol levels as it increases "good" (HDL) cholesterol. That's important because scientists think that increased levels of good HDL cholesterol protect against blood vessel disease and heart attack.

Slowly digested low-GI foods help to control blood-sugar levels in people with diabetes.

3

DIABETES AND CARBOHYDRATES

*D*IABETES IS A chronic condition in which the blood contains too much sugar. Normally, when we eat carbohydrate foods, our bodies break them down into a form that we can absorb and which our cells can use. This breaking-down process is digestion, the end product of which is blood glucose. (Digestion actually starts in the mouth as we chew our food and amylase, the digestive enzyme in saliva, is incorporated into the food.) Most digestion, however, takes place in the small intestine where enzymes break the large starch molecules down into simpler molecules. The resulting simple sugars (glucose, fructose, and galactose) are absorbed from the small intestine into the bloodstream.

To keep blood-sugar levels normal, we need the right amount of the hormone insulin. Insulin drives the sugar out of the blood and into the body's muscles, where it is used to provide energy for the body. If there isn't enough insulin or if the insulin doesn't do its job properly, we develop diabetes, of which there are two main types:

Type 1, or insulin-dependent, diabetes mellitus is most commonly diagnosed during childhood. In this type of diabetes, the pancreas doesn't produce enough insulin and a person needs multiple insulin injections every day to replace this deficit. Since the amount of insulin injected is prescribed, it's important for the person to regulate food intake to maintain a balanced blood-sugar level.

Although children and teenagers with type 1 diabetes are insulin-dependent, there are many steps they can take to reduce disease symptoms and complications.

Type 2, or non insulin-dependent, diabetes mellitus usually occurs in people over forty, although, as we mentioned earlier, the disease is now beginning to appear in younger people who are sedentary and overweight. People with type 2 diabetes can still make their own insulin, but either don't produce enough of it or produce insulin that doesn't work effectively. Exercise and eating a healthy diet is all that some people with type 2 diabetes have to do to keep their blood-sugar levels within the normal range, while other people may need to take medication or insulin injections.

Food for Thought

CARBOHYDRATES INCLUDE STARCHY foods, such as bread, cookies, potatoes, breakfast cereals, pasta, rice, and noodles, plus all the foods that contain natural or added sugar, such as fruit, milk, ice cream, jelly, chocolate, soft drinks, and candy.

No matter which type of diabetes your child has, there are many steps you can take to reduce disease symptoms and complications. That's what this book is all about.

■

The dietary guidelines for children with diabetes are the same as those for all children and teenagers.

■

◀ 4 ▶

WHAT TYPE OF CARBOHYDRATE?

*T*HANKS TO RESEARCH on the glycemic index, we now know that even people with diabetes can enjoy foods containing added sugar (in moderation, of course) as part of a healthy diet. Sugar itself has only an intermediate-GI value, which means that it has a moderate effect on blood-sugar levels compared with other carbohydrate foods. In fact, many sugar-containing foods, such as yogurt and flavored milk, actually have low-GI values and raise blood-sugar levels less than some refined wheat products.

You may be familiar with the carbohydrate exchange system that for many years has helped people with diabetes determine how much carbohydrate they can eat. (It has also been used extensively in the past in some weight loss programs.) The glycemic index research, however, has scientifically proven that this system is flawed, because the exchange system assumes that equal amounts of different carbohydrate foods have similar effects on blood-sugar levels. That's wrong. The change in blood sugar after one exchange of cornflakes, for example, is very different than after one exchange of apple.

Although the carbohydrate exchange system is a helpful guide to carbohydrate quantity, remember its limitations when it comes to predicting the impact of foods on your blood-sugar levels.

FOUR TIPS FOR CHOOSING CARBOHYDRATES

- Use standard household measures, such as ounces and cups to measure portions; the serving sizes listed on food labels aren't necessarily the amounts your child should eat.
- Your child should eat regular meals and snacks based on low-GI foods.
- Choose your child's carbohydrate from a wide variety of sources—both starch and sugar foods.
- Use the GI tables to choose the most suitable carbohydrate for your child. Aim to include at least one low-GI food in every meal and snack. (You'll find the GI Table on page 131.)

■

The glycemic index is a ranking of carbohydrate foods based on their immediate effect on blood-sugar levels.

■

◀ 5 ▶

SOURCES OF CARBOHYDRATE

At the beginning of this book we explained that carbohydrate is the fuel our bodies like best. Carbohydrate is important for children because it gives them the energy they need every day to play, study, and take part in sports.

Breads and cereals, vegetables, and fruits are all sources of carbohydrate. Milk products also contain carbohydrate in the form of milk sugar, or lactose, which is the first carbohydrate we consume as babies.

Some foods contain a large amount of carbohydrate (cereals, potatoes, and legumes are good examples), while other foods, such as carrots and broccoli and salad vegetables, are very dilute sources and don't provide nearly enough carbohydrate for our high carbohydrate diet. So, as nutritious as salads can be, they aren't meals on their own and need to be complemented with a carbohydrate food, such as whole grain bread or pasta.

◀ 6 ▶

WHY WE NEED MORE CARBOHYDRATE

MOST EXPERTS AGREE that breakfast, lunch, dinner, and in-between snack foods should be low in fat and high in carbohydrate. And when it comes to choosing the best fuel for vigorous and extended physical activity—whether it's sports or play—again, carbohydrate is the best choice. Studies show that a balanced carbohydrate meal enhances memory and learning; in fact, children's scores on classroom tests are higher if they consume healthy carbohydrates for breakfast.

In addition, carbohydrate and fat have a reciprocal relationship in our diets: if we eat more high carbohydrate foods they tend to displace the high-fat foods from our diet. And when carbohydrates (such as a breakfast of Special K, skim milk, and fruit, instead of a chocolate doughnut) displace saturated and trans fats, they improve the diet's overall nutritional quality. In fact, carbohydrate should be the main source of calories in our food—not fat.

A healthy, balanced diet for children contains a wide variety of foods.

CARBOHYDRATES AND INSULIN

THE PANCREAS IS a vital organ near the stomach, and its main job is to produce the hormone insulin. Carbohydrate stimulates the secretion of insulin more than any other component of food. The slow absorption of the carbohydrate in our food means that the pancreas doesn't have to work so hard and needs to produce less insulin. If the pancreas is overstimulated over a long period of time, it may become "exhausted" and type 2 diabetes can develop in genetically susceptible people. Even without diabetes, high-insulin levels are undesirable because they increase the risk of heart disease.

Unfortunately, over time, we have begun to eat more "refined" foods and fewer "whole" foods. This new way of eating has brought with it higher blood-sugar levels after a meal and higher insulin responses, as well. Though our bodies do need insulin for carbohydrate metabolism, high levels of the hormone have a profound effect on the development of many diseases. In fact, medical experts now believe that high insulin levels are one of the key factors responsible for heart disease and hypertension. Insulin influences the way we metabolize foods, determining whether we burn fat or carbohydrate to meet our energy needs and ultimately determining whether we store fat in our bodies.

◀ 7 ▶

THE GLYCEMIC INDEX: SOME BACKGROUND

*T*HE GLYCEMIC INDEX of foods is simply a ranking of foods based on their immediate effect on blood-sugar levels. To make a fair comparison, all foods are compared with a reference food, such as pure glucose, and are tested in equivalent carbohydrate amounts.

Today we know the glycemic index of hundreds of different food items—both generic and name-brand—that have been tested following a standardized testing method. The tables on pages 131–146 give the glycemic index of a range of common foods, including many tested at the University of Toronto and the University of Sydney.

HOW THE GLYCEMIC INDEX CAME TO BE

The glycemic index concept was first developed in 1981 by a team of scientists led by Dr. David Jenkins, a professor of nutrition at the University of Toronto, Canada, to help determine which foods were best for people with diabetes. At that time, the diet for people with diabetes was based on a system of carbohydrate exchanges or portions, which was complicated and not very logical. The carbohydrate exchange system assumed that all starchy foods produce the same effect on blood-sugar levels even though some earlier studies had already proven this was not correct. Jenkins was one of the first researchers to question this assumption and to investigate how real foods behave in the bodies of real people.

Jenkins's approach attracted a great deal of attention because it was so logical and systematic. He and his colleagues had tested a large number of common foods, and some of their results were surprising. Ice cream for example, despite its sugar content, had much less effect on blood sugar than some ordinary breads. Over the next fifteen years medical researchers and scientists around the world, including the authors of this book, tested the effect of many foods on blood-sugar levels and developed a new concept of classifying carbohydrates based on their glycemic index.

When we looked at the actual blood sugar responses to different foods in people we found that:

- Many complex carbohydrates, such as bread and potatoes, were actually digested and absorbed very quickly (contrary to popular opinion).
- Many sugar-containing foods were not the villains responsible for high blood sugars.

Carbohydrate foods that break down quickly during digestion have the highest GI values. The blood-glucose, or -sugar, response is fast and high. In other words the glucose in the bloodstream increases rapidly. Conversely, carbohydrates that break down slowly, releasing glucose gradually into the bloodstream, have low-GI values. An analogy might be the popular fable of the tortoise and the hare. The hare, just like high-GI foods, speeds away full steam ahead but loses the race to the tortoise with his slow and steady pace. Similarly, slow and steady low-GI foods produce a smooth blood-sugar curve without wild fluctuations.

For most people most of the time, the foods with low GI values have advantages over those with high-GI values. To see the effect of slow and fast carbohydrate on blood-sugar levels, see Figure 1, below.

Figure 1. The effect of pure glucose (50 grams) and lentils (50 grams carbohydrate portion) on blood-sugar levels.

THE GLYCEMIC INDEX IS:

- a scientifically proven guide to the actual effects of carbohydrate foods on blood-sugar levels, and
- an easy and effective way to eat a healthy diet and control fluctuations in blood sugar.

The glycemic index is a clinically proven tool in its applications to diabetes, appetite control, and reducing the risk of heart disease.

8

HOW WE MEASURE THE GLYCEMIC INDEX

THE SUBSTANCE THAT produces the greatest rise in blood-sugar levels is pure glucose itself. All other foods have less effect when fed in equal amounts of carbohydrate. The glycemic index of pure glucose is set at 100, and every other food is ranked on a scale from 0 to 100 according to its actual effect on blood-sugar levels.

We can't predict the glycemic index of a food from its composition or the glycemic index of related foods. To test the glycemic index, we need real people and real foods. There is no easy, inexpensive substitute test. Scientists always follow standardized methods so that results from one group of people can be directly compared with those of another group.

The most important point to note is that all foods are tested in equivalent carbohydrate amounts. For example, we test 100 grams of bread (about 3½ slices of sandwich bread) because that amount contains 50 grams of carbohydrate. Likewise, 60 grams of jelly beans (containing 50 grams of carbohydrate) is compared with the reference food. We know how much carbohydrate is in a food by consulting food composition tables, the manufacturer's data, or measuring it ourselves in the laboratory.

Scientists use just six steps to determine the glycemic index of a food. Simple as this may sound, it's actually quite a time consuming process. Here's how it works:

1. An amount of food containing 50 grams of carbohydrate is given to a volunteer to eat. For example, to test boiled spaghetti, the volunteer would be given 200 grams of spaghetti, which supplies 50 grams of carbohydrate (we work this out from food composition tables or by measuring the available carbohydrate)—50 grams of carbohydrate is equivalent to 3 tablespoons of pure glucose powder.
2. Over the next two hours (or three hours if the volunteer has diabetes), we take a sample of their blood every 15 minutes during the first hour and thereafter every 30 minutes. The blood-sugar level of these blood samples is measured in the laboratory and recorded.
3. The blood-sugar level is plotted on a graph and the area under the curve is calculated using a computer program (Figure 2, page 22.).
4. The volunteer's response to spaghetti (or whatever food is being tested) is compared with his or her blood-sugar response to 50 grams of pure glucose (the reference food).
5. The reference food is tested on two or three separate occasions and an average value is calculated. This is done to reduce the effect of day-to-day variation in blood-sugar responses.

6. The average glycemic index value found in eight to ten people is the GI value of that food.

GLUCOSE (reference food) — 100%

SPAGHETTI (test food) — 41%

Blood-Sugar Levels vs. time (1 hour, 2 hours)

Figure 2.

GI Ranges

Low GI	0–55
Intermediate GI	56–69
High GI	70 or higher

PART 2

THE GLYCEMIC INDEX AND YOUR CHILD

9

LOW-GI DIETS FOR CHILDREN

It's easy to incorporate low-GI foods into a child's diet and rewarding to watch them reap the benefits. It usually just means making a few substitutions, such as those shown on page 26. Ideally, you should aim to swap at least half of the high-GI foods that you give children for low-GI choices. For example, you could change the type of bread or breakfast cereal your child eats and serve pasta or legumes more often. And don't forget milk and dairy foods.

Remember that it isn't necessary to serve children only low-GI foods. On the contrary, meals usually consist of a variety of foods, and eating a low-GI food with a high-GI food produces an intermediate GI meal. Here are three ways to make serving low-GI foods easier:

♦ Become familiar with the different types of low-GI choices available.

- Have low-GI foods available in the pantry and refrigerator.
- Experiment with new foods and recipes.

Try to include at least one low-GI food per meal per day.

Low-GI Substitutes

HIGH-GI FOOD	LOW-GI ALTERNATIVE
Bread, whole-wheat or white	Whole-grain pumpernickel, sourdough, 100% stone-ground whole-wheat, whole-wheat pita, sourdough rye
Processed breakfast cereal	Unrefined cereal, such as rolled oats or a low-GI processed cereal, like All Bran™
Plain cookies and crackers	Cookies made with dried fruit and whole grains, such as oats
Cakes and muffins	Make them with fruit, oats, whole grains
White potato	Substitute with new or sweet potatoes, or other starches, such as corn, pasta, and legumes
Sticky or parboiled rice	Try Basmati or Uncle Ben's Converted rice, pearled barley, or noodles
Tropical fruits	Temperate-climate fruits, such as bananas, apples, peaches, and nectarines

10

WHO BENEFITS FROM LOW-GI FOODS?

*W*E ALL DO! The slow digestion and gradual rise and fall in blood-sugar levels after eating a low-GI food reduces the secretion of the hormone insulin into the blood. High-insulin levels are undesirable because they increase our risk of heart disease, diabetes, and obesity. Reducing this risk is why low-GI foods benefit everyone—people with and without diabetes. These facts are no exaggeration. They're confirmed by many studies published in prestigious journals around the world.

LOW-GI/HIGH-GI CHOICES

A food is neither good nor bad based on its glycemic index value. For example, if a food is high in fat, it's not a good idea to eat it regularly just because it has a low-GI value. By the same token, we shouldn't demonize low-fat, high-GI foods like some types of potatoes. The truth is, eating a potato is far better than eating a food loaded with saturated fat, even if its glycemic index value is low.

Consider the GI value of a food in conjunction with its fat, fiber and salt content—not by itself.

Food for Thought

CHILDREN HAVE DIFFERENT nutritional requirements at different ages. That's why, if you have a child with diabetes, you'll need to review and adjust her diet with the help of a dietitian.

THE FOOD PYRAMID FOR CHILDREN

*S*CHOOL-AGE CHILDREN have changing energy needs due to their growth rate, body size, and physical-activity level. All children need at least the minimum number of servings from each of the five food groups every day. Older, larger, and more active children will require the maximum number of servings, which will give their bodies the 1,800 to 2,200 calories they require for proper growth and good health.

THE FOOD PYRAMID FOR CHILDREN AGES 2 TO 6

- **Fats, Oils, Sweets** (USE SPARINGLY)
- **Milk, Yogurt, Cheese** — 2–3 SERVINGS
- **Meat, Poultry, Fish, Dried Beans, Eggs, Nuts** — 2–3 SERVINGS
- **Vegetables** — 3–4 SERVINGS
- **Fruits** — 2–3 SERVINGS
- **Bread, Cereal, Rice, Pasta** — 6–9 SERVINGS

Is Your Child Getting Enough Water?

Water Requirements	Ounces/Lb./Day
0–3 mos.	1.2–2.5
4–6 mos.	2.0–2.3
7–12 mos.	1.8–2.0
1 year	1.8–2.0
2 years	1.7–1.9
6 years	1.4–1.3

■

If children learn to combine regular physical activity with healthy low-GI eating early in their lives, they will develop healthy lifestyle habits that may continue into adulthood.

■

◀ 12 ▶

BLOOD SUGAR AND EXERCISE

GOOD HEALTH, A reasonable body weight, and good blood-sugar levels are all easier to achieve if children exercise, because their insulin will work better.

If they get additional exercise or take part in activities outside their normal routine, children may need to eat extra carbohydrates as a precaution to prevent their blood-sugar levels from dropping too low. Just how much extra carbohydrate they'll need will depend on their fitness level, the type and length of activity, and the amount of effort they're expending. As a rough guide, one extra serving of carbohydrate is suggested for every hour of strenuous activity. Generally, the more strenuous and the longer the duration of the exercise, the more additional carbohydrate they will require.

Your child's usual insulin dose (if any) and food intake covers normal play activities—even quite strenuous ones.

APPROPRIATE BLOOD-SUGAR LEVELS

If your child's blood sugar is less than 180 mg/dl before exercise, she may need to eat extra carbohydrates before, during, and after exercise to prevent hypoglycemia. (Mg/dl is a unit of measurement for the concentration of sugar in a given quantity of blood.)

If your child's blood sugar is more than 270 mg/dl and ketones are present in her urine before exercise, ask her to postpone exercise until her overall control has improved. Otherwise, exercise may actually increase her blood-sugar level further. (Ketones are a product of fat breakdown that occurs when there isn't enough insulin available. Without adequate insulin, the body isn't able to use its preferred fuel—glucose—so it uses fat instead.)

Since everyone responds to exercise differently, your child may need to eat extra carbohydrates before and/or during and/or after exercise, and the quantity she needs may also vary.

You and your child will learn from experience what works best for her; at first, monitoring her blood sugar before, during, and after exercise will give both of you the best indication of how her body responds.

SUSTAINING BLOOD-SUGAR LEVELS DURING EXERCISE

- If children eat immediately before exercising, they should select foods with a high glycemic index, such as sugar wafers, candy, granola bars, or a white bread sandwich.
- When kids eat 1 or 2 hours before exercising,

they should choose low-GI foods, such as yogurt, a sandwich made from low-GI bread, low-GI cereals, low-GI fruits, or milkshakes.
- If children need to eat during prolonged exercise (over an hour), they need to choose foods with a high glycemic index that they can eat on the run. Liquids—sports drinks—may be best because they meet fuel and fluid requirements at the same time.
- If kids eat between events throughout the day (such as at bike races or a day at the beach) they should eat a combination of low- and high-GI foods. It is generally appropriate to decrease the usual insulin dose (if any) by 10 percent as well, so that they don't need to eat too much food.
- If children require additional foods to restore blood-sugar levels after exercise, they should choose high-GI foods, such as rice cakes, white bread, watermelon, or a high-GI cereal, such as Rice Krispies or corn flakes. They need to drink plenty of water, too, or select high-GI fluids to meet both carbohydrate and fluid needs at the same time.

Exercise means being active every day— whether it's playing a sport, taking part in an active hobby, or walking the dog after school.

◀ 13 ▶

BLOOD-SUGAR GUIDELINES

*I*N ORDER TO maintain a healthy weight, children of all ages need to strike a balance between eating a well-balanced diet based on low-GI foods and getting enough exercise. Low-GI foods not only help your child maintain blood-sugar control, but they're also more sustaining and can make her feel fuller longer, compared with foods with a high-GI value.

To make sure that they eat well and exercise regularly, all kids should:

- Limit high-fat foods, such as chocolate, cookies, fried foods, burgers, potato chips, and cake.
- Keep in contact with their health professional. As they lose weight, their diabetes team should review their insulin doses.
- Do something active everyday. Increasing physical activity doesn't have to mean vigorous exercise. It simply means spending less time lying around.

- Incorporate exercise into their daily routine. There are lots of options, from team sports to aerobics classes, swimming, or gym workouts. If youngsters want to do something less structured, they can walk, jog, cycle, or inline skate.

Being more active makes kids look better and feel better. Honest!

Food for Thought

STUDIES SHOW THAT people who take more than 12,500 steps a day don't gain weight over the long term, no matter what they eat. Children can measure how many steps they take in a single day by using a pedometer.

◀ 14 ▶

HANDLING LOW BLOOD SUGAR

*H*YPOGLYCEMIA OCCURS WHEN there are low levels of sugar in the blood, usually below 55 to 70 mg/dl. Low blood sugar may be caused by:

- taking too much insulin;
- exercising vigorously without eating extra carbohydrate;
- missing or delaying meals; or
- not eating an adequate amount of carbohydrate food.

How children feel when their blood sugar is low varies from child to child. Common symptoms are excessive sweating, tiredness, drowsiness, irritability, dizziness, shaking, headache, and blurred vision.

■

Learn the signs of low blood sugar and act quickly. If these dips happen often, contact your doctor or diabetes educator so they can review your child's insulin dose, if any, and diet.

■

WHAT TO DO ABOUT LOW BLOOD SUGAR

To combat hypoglycemia, your child should:

- eat a quickly absorbed (high GI) carbohydrate food that's easy to eat or drink (jellybeans, regular soda, Gatorade, orange juice). The food will immediately increase blood-sugar levels. If she sees no improvement, your child should eat more high-GI food after five minutes have passed;
- follow the above guideline by eating an intermediate or low-GI food (bread, cookies, fruit, milk) ten to fifteen minutes after to a) ensure that her blood-sugar level remains within the normal range longer and b) prevent the hypo from recurring;
- always carry high-GI foods or glucose tablets to treat hypoglycemia;
- remember that the extra foods she eats for low blood sugar are *extra* and should not be subtracted from her next meal or snack;
- try to determine why the hypoglycemia occurred, in order to help prevent it from happening again. Most hypoglycemic episodes are preventable but some occur for no apparent reason.

■

Don't leave someone with hypoglycemia unattended until they are feeling better.

■

COPING WITH LOW BLOOD SUGAR AT NIGHT

Hypoglycemia can occur at night. Most of the time, though, children wake when they're experiencing low blood sugar, or at least they become restless enough that their parents wake up. Sometimes, however, children sleep soundly through a blood sugar drop and the body self-corrects and over-compensates, which shows up as a high blood sugar reading the next morning.

MINIMIZING THE RISK OF NIGHTTIME HYPOGLYCEMIA

You can help to reduce the risk of low blood sugar at night by asking your child to:

- eat a low-GI bedtime snack (such as a glass of milk or no-sugar-added hot chocolate and three Social Tea biscuits or one slice of toast), even if the evening blood sugar test is high;
- never skip the bedtime snack, even if the evening blood sugar test is high;
- test blood-sugar levels before bed, once your doctor has helped you determine her appropriate pre-bed level. Your child may need some extra carbohydrate.

Food for Thought

HAVE A REGISTERED Dietitian evaluate your child's normal calorie intake to make sure that it's adequate. Because a child's energy needs vary with age and physical activity levels, an ongoing nutritional assessment can help with blood sugar control.

◀ 15 ▶

SICK DAY HYPOGLYCEMIA

*H*AVING A SICK child can be hard enough, but a sick child with diabetes means that you need to be extra vigilant about blood sugar levels and appetite. Here are some guidelines.

IF BLOOD-SUGAR READINGS ARE GREATER THAN 270 MG/DL:

Serve your child low calorie fluids, such as water or decaffeinated diet drinks. You may also offer slightly smaller portions of carbohydrate foods while the sugar remains high since you're monitoring the readings more frequently. Don't omit carbohydrate foods altogether.

IF BLOOD-SUGAR READINGS ARE LESS THAN 270 MG/DL:

Serve your child some form of carbohydrate. Choosing foods from the intermediate GI range (or combining low-GI foods with high-GI foods) will help sustain blood-sugar levels while your child has a reduced appetite. Try serving:

plain toast	ice cream	stewed fruit
dry crackers	milkshakes	fruit juices
cookies	soup	potato chips

If your child's appetite is poor, he or she should frequently eat or sip intermediate to high-GI foods. (It may be easier for your child to eat smaller amounts more often.) Try offering these foods:

a sweetened soft drink	sweetened jelly
jellybeans	Jello
Gatorade	ices or ice pops
lollipops	pudding

If your child has diarrhea associated with gastroenteritis, you *must* dilute sweet fluids with water (four parts water to one part soft drink). Avoid serving your child full-strength sweet fluid, since that may actually worsen the diarrhea. Some salty fluids, such as soup broths or tomato juice, may also help your child rehydrate.

> **Food for Thought**
>
> **OCCASIONALLY CHECK YOUR** child's blood-sugar readings at 2:00 or 3:00 A.M. This early-morning check is especially important if your child is sick, has eaten poorly over the course of the day, has been unusually active, or if you suspect nighttime hypoglycemia.

GENERAL SICK-DAY GUIDELINES

Your child is likely to get coughs and colds and all the normal childhood illnesses. Unfortunately, sickness can make diabetes hard to manage, and lack of appetite is partly to blame. It's essential to monitor blood sugars closely during an illness.

ALWAYS GIVE INSULIN TO KIDS WHO TAKE IT

When children are sick, their liver is still producing (perhaps overproducing) glucose to maintain blood-sugar levels. Insulin is essential in order to manage this output. To maintain blood glucose control:

- Monitor blood-sugar levels every two hours.
- Test for ketones in the urine throughout the day. Your child may need extra insulin (if used) if ketones are present.
- Continue to serve some form of carbohydrate and make sure your child drinks plenty of fluids.

■

If you're ever in doubt when caring for a sick child with diabetes, call your diabetes doctor or educator for additional advice.

■

PART 3

FOOD BASICS

16

CEREALS AND GRAIN FOODS

TODAY, CEREAL AND grains are major sources of energy and protein for people all over the world, but they weren't part of the diet that humankind evolved on millions of years ago. As human populations grew, resources of mammals, fish, and birds became depleted. It's only been over the last ten thousand years that we've begun to rely more on cereals for food—with consequent developments in processing.

Unprocessed cereals and grains are naturally slowly digested foods. In early times, they were roughly ground between stones, which broke the outer seed husk but left much of the grain intact and produced a coarse meal. Today, cereal processing includes milling the grain into a fine flour, then popping, toasting, flaking, and extrusion cooking to make cakes, breads, cookies, snack products, and breakfast cereals.

One of the nutritional implications of this dietary change has been an increase in the GI value, because modern processing methods transform the low-GI carbohydrate of cereal grains to high-GI foods. In other words, because of the processing (or refinement) of whole grains, our bodies have much less work to do to digest them into blood sugar (glucose) and dump them into the bloodstream.

To help your child eat a low-GI diet, serve less-processed cereal products and whole grain cereals. Hint: The higher the fiber content, the more intact the grains are. Aim for 5 grams of fiber or more per serving.

PASTA

Most children love pasta. And not only is it good to eat, it's good to eat it often because whether you choose penne or spaghetti or fettuccine, you are choosing one of nature's naturally low-GI foods.

Most pasta is made from semolina (finely cracked wheat), which is milled from very hard wheat with a high-protein content. A stiff dough, made by mixing the semolina with water, is forced through a die and dried. There is very little disruption of the starch granule during this process and the strong protein-starch interactions inhibit starch gelatinization. The dense consistency also makes the pasta resistant to disruption in the small intestine and contributes to the final low-glycemic index—even pasta made from fine flour (instead of semolina) has a relatively low-glycemic index. There's some evidence that thicker pasta has a lower glycemic index than thin types because of its dense consistency and perhaps because it cooks more slowly. (It's also less likely to be overcooked.) The addition of egg to fresh pasta lowers the GI value by increasing the protein content: Higher protein levels slow stomach emptying, because only about 60 percent of the protein gets broken down; the rest goes into storage as fat.

Italians eat their pasta *al dente* which literally means "to the tooth." It must be slightly firm and offer some resistance when you're chewing it. Not only does al dente pasta taste better than soft, soggy pasta, but it also has a lower GI value, because overcooking pasta increases starch gelatinization (or swelling) and boosts its glycemic index.

Our books *The New Glucose Revolution* and *The New Glucose Revolution Life Plan* have many recipes that your whole family will enjoy.

RICE

Rice is an ideal accompaniment to spicy foods. Milling rice removes the bran and germ, which results in a considerable nutrient loss. Brown rice is a better source of B vitamins, minerals and fiber; be sure to vary your family's diet to include both brown and white rice. And look for other lower GI rices, including Uncle Ben's converted or Basmati rice, in your supermarket.

BREAD

One of the most important changes you can make to lower the GI value of your children's diet is to choose a low-GI bread when making toast, sandwiches, or snacks.

Choose dense breads that contain a lot of whole grains: If the fibrous seed coat of cereal grains is intact, it acts as a physical barrier to slow down starch digestion. Pumpernickel is a true whole grain bread—it's made from whole rye grains.

Other low-GI breads include sourdough and stone-ground flour breads (types that don't contain any enriched wheat flour). The acids in sourdough breads may reduce the glycemic index—the acids that result from fermentation of the starch and sugars are believed to lower GI values by slowing down stomach emptying. To add more bread to your child's meals, read our sandwich suggestions for snacks and school lunches on pages 96 and 105.

If you're making your own bread, you can add your own GI lowering ingredients, such as linseed, flaxseed, rolled oats, cornmeal, oat bran, barley meal, cracked wheat, and wheat berries.

◀ 17 ▶

VEGETABLES

*Y*OUR CHILDREN CAN eat most vegetables without thinking about their glycemic index. Most are so low in carbohydrate that they have no measurable effect on blood-sugar levels, but they still provide valuable amounts of fiber, vitamins, and minerals. Higher carbohydrate vegetables include potato, sweet potato, corn, and peas. Among these, corn and sweet potato are the lower GI choices. Pumpkin, carrots, peas, and beets contain some carbohydrate but a half-cup serving contains so little that these foods don't raise blood-sugar levels significantly.

Salad vegetables, such as tomatoes, lettuce, cucumber, peppers, and onions also have so little carbohydrate that it's impossible to test their glycemic index values. In generous serving sizes, they won't have any effect on blood sugars. Think of them as "free" foods that are full of healthful micronutrients.

◀ 18 ▶

FRUIT

*N*ot only does fruit make an ideal snack, you can transform it into a tasty, sweet dessert quickly and easily. Fruit contains carbohydrate, fiber, vitamins (such as vitamin C and beta-carotene), and minerals. Most fresh fruit contains vitamin C, so all of us—not just our children—should eat it every day, preferably whole, rather than as juice.

Most fruits have low-GI values thanks to the low glycemic index of fructose (a major sugar in fruit). The presence of viscous fiber, such as pectin and acids (which may slow down stomach emptying), also help keep the glycemic index low.

- Fruits with the lowest GI values tend to be those grown in temperate climates, such as apples, pears, citrus, peaches, plums, cherries, and all berries.

- The more acidic the fruit, the lower its glycemic index; for example, grapefruit's glycemic index is 25.
- Tropical fruits, such as melons, pineapples and bananas, have intermediate-GI values.

◀ 19 ▶

DAIRY FOODS

*Y*OU SHOULD ENCOURAGE your children to eat dairy foods throughout their childhood and beyond. Not only are dairy foods an important source of calcium but they also have low-GI values. Dairy foods also provide energy, protein, carbohydrate, vitamin B_2, and important fat-soluble vitamins, such as vitamins A and D.

If for some reason your child is allergic to cow's milk, try a lactose-free milk or suitable calcium-fortified soy substitute (approximately 180 mg of calcium per 4 ounces). The soy drinks that we have tested have low-GI values—similar to cow's milk. The good news is that most children will outgrow a cow's milk allergy by five years of age.

Calcium helps build and maintain strong bones and teeth and has other important nerve and muscle functions. Milk, yogurt, ice cream, pudding, and custard are all excellent low-GI sources of calcium. Cheese, although a good source of calcium, is considered a source of protein rather than carbohydrate, and contains no lactose.

◀ 20 ▶

MEAT AND MEAT ALTERNATIVES

*P*ROTEINS ARE THE body's building blocks, so we need to eat a variety of protein foods from animal or plant sources to create, maintain, and renew our body cells. Children and teenagers, because they are growing, need more protein in relation to their body weight than adults do because they are building new body cells.

- Red meat, chicken, pork, and fish are important sources of protein and micronutrients, such as iron. They don't contain carbohydrate so they don't have a GI value. Choose lean meats where possible; there are now many trim cuts available. Serve *infrequently* such fatty processed meats as sausage, frankfurters, chicken nuggets, and salami.
- Include fish in the family meals at least once a week, especially tuna or salmon, which are high in heart-healthy omega-3 essential fatty acids.

- Legumes, such as split peas, baked beans, and lentils provide protein, vitamin B, and iron, as does meat, but legumes are also excellent low GI sources of carbohydrate. Try to incorporate them in family meals at least once a week.

Natural Peanut Butter

NATURAL PEANUT BUTTER is a high-protein, nutrient-dense food. It contains fiber, iron, and heart-healthy monounsaturated fat. Peanut butter and all-fruit jelly on whole grain bread is a great breakfast, lunch, or snack that requires little time or skill to prepare! And just for variety, you can try other nut butters, such as cashew, almond, and soy.

◀ 21 ▶

FATS AND OILS

ALTHOUGH FAT DOESN'T directly affect blood-sugar levels, it isn't something that you can ignore. The fat that children (and all of us) eat affects their body weight, cholesterol levels, risk of diabetic complications, and odds of developing poor health from everyday diseases such as obesity, heart disease, and even cancer.

Although a low-fat diet is *not recommended* for very young children, once a child is older than five, it's fine for them to eat low-fat products. If your child is overweight, limiting fat intake will likely help, but you should only do this under the guidance of a registered dietitian.

It's important to consider what type of fat your child eats. For example, polyunsaturated fats, such as margarine and vegetable oils, and monounsaturated fats, such as olive and canola oils, are preferable to saturated fats, such as butter and fatty meats. In fact, we all should limit our saturated fat intake. It's particularly important for children to avoid saturated fat because the changes in blood vessels that lead to heart disease begin in childhood. You'll find a list of high-fat foods on this page.

Food for Thought

The omega-3 fats found in fish are important sources of healthy fat for adults as well as children, so try to serve fish, such as salmon and white albacore tuna, regularly.

High-Fat Foods to Watch Out for:

- Butter
- Cakes, cookies
- Cheese
- Chicken nuggets
- Whole milk (Children under age two should be given whole milk.)
- Corn chips
- Creamy soups, sauces, and desserts
- Doughnuts
- French fries
- Ice creams
- Most milkshakes
- Pastries
- Pies
- Pizza with meat and cheese toppings
- Potato chips
- Sausages
- Solid cooking fats and cooking margarines; white fat on beef, lamb, pork, vegetable shortening

22

SUGAR

CHILDREN NATURALLY ENJOY sweet foods. Sweetness is not a learned taste; in fact, it could be said that we're all born with "a sweet tooth." Not only is our first food—breast milk—sweet, but also infants smile when offered a sweet solution, as they reject sour and bitter tastes.

Did you know that a balanced diet should include some fat and sugar? Studies over the past decade have found that high-sugar diets are no less nutritious than diets containing lower amounts of sugar: When we restrict sugar, we frequently eat more fat, and the most popular fatty foods are poor sources of nutrients. In some cases, high-sugar diets may have higher micronutrient contents, because sugar is often used to sweeten some very nutritious foods, such as yogurt, breakfast cereals, and milk.

Today, glycemic index researchers have tested hundreds of real foods on real people, and the results are surprising.

Sugar is not the dietary demon that it was once made out to be. Many Americans, though, eat far too much of it. Sixteen percent of our average daily caloric intake comes from sweeteners (health experts recommend 6 to 10 percent). That's why you need to look at your child's diet and adjust her sugar intake accordingly. Your child can enjoy sugar and foods containing sugar *in moderation* as part of a balanced low-GI diet.

> ### Food for Thought
>
> **IT'S NOT A** good idea for children—or any of us—to eat an excess of artificially sweetened products. Many of these products, such as diet sodas and sugar-free candies and sweets, are simply flavored fillers and provide few, if any, nutrients. It is nutritionally unwise to allow children to fill up on calorie-free, nutrient-free foods—serve them nutrient-packed foods instead.

WHAT EXACTLY IS "MODERATE INTAKE"?

A moderate intake of refined sugar for a child is about 6 teaspoons a day. Keep in mind that we're talking about the sugar found in foods, such as all non-diet soft drinks, breakfast cereals, candy, ice cream, cookies, jelly, and syrups. Staying within this amount of sugar can make your child's diet more enjoyable without compromising her blood-sugar control.

A MODERATE-SUGAR MENU

This child's menu provides 45 grams of refined sugar (about 3½ tablespoons) and 1,700 calories (29 percent of energy from fat, 54 percent from carbohydrate and 17 percent from protein).

Breakfast
½ cup Special K with 6 ozs. 1% milk
½ cup strawberries
1 teaspoon sugar

Mid-morning snack
4 ozs. unsweetened applesauce
15 Teddy Grahams

Lunch
Ham and cheese sandwich on multigrain bread with lettuce and tomato
1 cup grapes
2 Chips Ahoy chocolate chip cookies

After-school snack
6 ozs. 1% milk
6 Social Tea biscuits

Dinner
1 cup spaghetti with ½ cup meat sauce
½ cup steamed French cut green beans
½ cup Snack Pack tapioca pudding

Bedtime snack
- 1 slice cinnamon raisin toast with butter or margarine
- 4 ozs. 1% milk

Fast-Acting Carbohydrates

IT IS ABSOLUTELY essential to serve refined sugars or "fast-acting" carbohydrates:

- during periods of hypoglycemia (low blood-sugar levels);
- when your child is ill and has little or no appetite;
- immediately before exercise or strenuous activity; and
- as a treat or on a special occasion.

Food for Thought

"CARBOHYDRATE MODIFIED" SUGAR alcohols, such as sorbitol, mannitol, and xylitol, often produce a laxative effect if you eat too much of them.

PART 4

AGE-SPECIFIC INFORMATION FOR DIABETIC CHILDREN

23

BABIES

*B*ABIES WITH DIABETES should be breast-fed if possible. Although infants should dictate how much they eat, you should monitor their blood sugars routinely. If it's not possible to breast-feed, offer your baby an infant formula at least every three to four hours.

Until your baby is twelve months old, milk should be her main drink. When your baby is about seven months old, you can introduce whole cows' milk in small quantities as custard, pudding, yogurt, or on cereal. From twelve months, when your baby is eating a varied diet, you can give her whole cows' milk as her main drink. Encourage your baby to eat dairy foods because they're an important source of calcium and have low-GI values—a big advantage when you're trying to optimize your baby's blood sugar control.

You can begin introducing your child to solids (including low-GI foods) anytime from five to six months—when your baby is ready. By twelve months she should be enjoying the family meal with you and drinking whole cows' milk from a cup. (Your whole family can enjoy delicious low-GI meals: Our books *The New Glucose Revolution* and *The New Glucose Revolution Life Plan* contain hundreds of recipes, and meal and snack ideas that your whole family will enjoy.)

> ### Food for Thought
>
> **A WORD ABOUT TODDLER TANTRUMS:** Tantrums are common among independent toddlers. But sometimes it's difficult to determine whether a toddler is irritable because of hypoglycemia or the "terrible twos." When in doubt, remember that it's potentially more dangerous not to treat hypoglycemia in a young child.

Recommended daily quantities of food in baby's first year

AGE IN MONTHS	FOOD GROUP	FOOD	SUGGESTED DAILY AMOUNT
5–6	Dairy	Breast milk or infant formula	On demand (maximum intake 36 ozs. in 24 hours)
	Grains	Pureed/strained iron-fortified cereal: rice, barley, or oatmeal	Start with 1 tablespoon per feeding and gradually increase to 3 tablespoons/ 2 servings a day
7–9	Dairy	Breast milk or infant formula	On demand (maximum intake 36 ozs. in 24 hours)
	Grains	Pureed/strained iron-fortified cereal: rice, barley, oatmeal, Cream of Wheat, farina. Add dry low-GI toast and crackers (not cookies)	1–3 tablespoons/ 2 servings a day
	Vegetables	Strained carrots, green beans, green peas, squash, sweet potatoes	Start with 1 tablespoon per feeding, increase to 2 tablespoons per feeding 2 servings a day. Add one new food every 5–6 days
	Fruit	Start fruits after vegetables. Single strained fruit (pear, peaches) or mashed banana; unsweetened fruit juice in a cup	2–3 tablespoons/ 2 servings a day
	Meat	Start meats after vegetables and fruits. Strained beef, liver, veal, turkey, chicken, lamb, or pork	2 tablespoons per feeding/1–2 servings a day

THE NEW GLUCOSE REVOLUTION

AGE IN MONTHS	FOOD GROUP	FOOD	SUGGESTED DAILY AMOUNT
10–12	Dairy	Breast milk or infant formula. May also add soft cheese, pudding, and, occasionally, custard	On demand (maximum intake intake 36 ozs. in 24 hours) from a bottle or cup
	Grains	Continue with high iron cereals and low GI breads. Avoid cookies and cakes	1/2 cup/2 servings a day
	Vegetables	Slowly begin to increase variety. All vegetables should be cooked; may be mashed or left whole in small soft pieces. Vegetables may be spoon-fed or eaten as finger foods.	1/4 cup/2 servings a day
	Fruit	Gradually increase variety. Avoid all fruits with seeds, pits, or thick skins	3 servings a day (limit fruit juice to 4 ozs. per day)
	High Protein Foods	In addition to previously mentioned choices—all of which should be appropriately cooked, ground, pureed, mashed, or flaked—cooked egg yolk (no whites) and fish may also be offered.	1–2 servings a day

Source: *Manual for Clinical Dietetics*, Fifth Edition, Chicago: The American Dietetic Association, 1996.

*It is recommended to prepare all the above listed foods at home and to avoid commercially prepared baby foods. Home preparation ensures greater nutritive value.

> ### Food for Thought
>
> **WHEN POSSIBLE, AVOID** feeding your children junior baby foods because of their limited nutritive value, limited variety, and high price.

Here is a list of foods that you *should not* feed infants less than one year old:

- Whole, low-fat, non-fat, or evaporated cow's milk
- Cereal in a bottle
- Cereal-egg-meat mixtures in jars
- Cookies, cakes, or sweet breads
- Vegetables seasoned with fat, salt, sugar, or other seasonings
- Strong-flavored vegetables
- Whole kernel corn
- Infant or homemade desserts, pies, or honey-fruit mixtures
- Fruits with seeds, pits, or thick skins
- Vegetable-meat or pasta-meat combinations
- Fatback, bacon
- Pork, sausages
- Broth, gravy
- Candy, nuts, or popcorn
- Fried foods
- Carbonated and sweetened beverages
- Regular tea

◀ 24 ▶

TODDLERS AND PRE-SCHOOLERS

Although toddlers like to explore and show their independence, they are still too young to understand their dietary needs. This lack of understanding can sometimes cause difficulties when children are with their friends, at playgroup or when grown-ups "spoil" them with too many treats. Among toddlers and pre-schoolers, picky eating and food fads are also common.

Toddlers don't eat much, simply because they don't need to eat much. Refusing food is also a way for them to express their newfound independence. That's why it's important not to fuss or pay her special attention, since a hungry toddler will never starve.

The trouble is, children with diabetes need to eat carbohydrates regularly to prevent hypoglycemia, so parents naturally become anxious. But bribing, bullying, and fussing usually only make matters worse. The best way to cope with food refusal is to try to avoid the whole situation in the first place. Allow your toddler to graze throughout the day according to her appetite rather than expecting her to eat meals at set times. Here are some other strategies to help defuse the situation:

Don't panic. Don't resort to circus tricks, since this may give your child the impression that if she refuses food, she'll get lots of attention.

Bargain calmly. Try to get the carbohydrate foods in first: "You can leave your egg if you eat your toast."

Try substituting. Substitute food that your toddler is refusing with another carbohydrate food that you know she likes. Offer only one alternative food each time though, or you could be starting a never-ending game of choices. Don't offer indulgent snack foods as alternatives.

Try finger foods and snacks. If your toddler still refuses to eat, leave finger foods (such as fruit pieces, crackers, or finger sandwiches) nearby so she can nibble as she plays.

Try distraction. Sitting your toddler on your lap and reading her a book can be a good distraction and may encourage her to eat.

Be prepared for low blood sugar. When all else fails, be prepared for hypoglycemia. If that happens, serve Gatorade or a soft drink. Just don't treat the low blood sugar with jelly beans or candy: Your child may interpret candy as a reward for not eating her meal, which would reinforce her food refusals.

WHEN YOUR CHILD CONTINUES TO REFUSE FOOD

You may need to reduce your child's insulin dose temporarily to minimize the risk of hypoglycemia and to reduce her tension and anxiety until she begins to eat more.

Remember, there's no single food that your toddler must eat. Encourage her to enjoy exploring new tastes and sensations in unchallenged and comfortable surroundings.

Try introducing new foods together with familiar foods that your toddler likes. Try offering them at several different meals and with other children who like to eat those foods. Never force her to eat, since too much pressure may only encourage her to refuse food. Respect your toddler's wishes if she says that she's full. Encourage her during mealtime so that she feels confident about trying new tastes.

Recommended Daily Quantities of Food for Todlers and Pre-Schoolers

FOOD GROUP	RECOMMENDED DAILY SERVINGS	RECOMMENDED SERVING SIZES 1-3 YRS.	4-5 YRS.
Bread (low GI)		1/4–1/2 slice	1 slice
Crackers (low GI)	≥ 6	2–3	4–6
Dry cereal (low GI)		1/4–1/3 cup	1/2 cup
Cooked cereal, rice, pasta (low GI)		1/4–1/3 cup	1/3 cup
Fruits and vegetables (low GI)	≥5	1/4–1/3 cup 1/2 piece	1/4–1/2 cup 1/2 piece
Milk, yogurt	≥ 3	1/2 cup (4 ozs.)	3/4 cup (6 ozs.)
Lean meat, fish, poultry		1–2 ozs.	2–3 ozs.
Cheese	≥ 2	1/2 oz.	3/4 oz.
Eggs		1	1
Dried peas, beans	1–3 Tbsp.	1–3 Tbsp.	
Margarine, butter, oil	3–4	1 tsp.	1 tsp.

Source: *Manual for Clinical Dietetics*, Fifth Edition, Chicago: The American Dietetic Association, 1996.

◀ 25 ▶

SCHOOL-AGE CHILDREN

Once they're at school, children with diabetes usually become more independent and start taking some responsibility for their own diabetes care. You should encourage this responsibility, although you should still continue to support and supervise your child. The majority of diabetic primary school children take two injections per day (if they do use insulin), pre-breakfast and pre-dinner. Since blood testing during the school day usually isn't required, children with diabetes can attend school without having to deal with the hassles of injections and finger pricks. Teachers, the school nurse, and other school staff should be fully educated and updated on your child's diabetes status.

LUNCH BOX IDEAS

At school, children compare lunch boxes and start trading and swapping what's inside. It's important that your child understand her diet and the carbohydrates she eats so that she can make appropriate lunch swaps. To make her more aware, involve her in preparing her school lunch. Pack enough foods to cover recess and lunch, and possibly extra snacks for sports or after-school activities.

Try to include an interesting selection of low-GI food choices each day and vary the contents regularly so she doesn't become bored. It's important to remember that most kids don't want to stand out from their peers, so the contents of your child's lunch box shouldn't look too different from her friends'. (For some nutritious, wholesome lunch ideas, see "The Low-GI Lunch Box" on pages 77–78 and "Lunches and Sandwich Fillers" on page 96.) Here are some hints for packing a lunch:

- Don't worry if your child selects the same foods for her lunch box everyday as long as her food choices are mainly healthy. She will let you know when she's bored and ready for more variety.
- Make sure that you pack enough carbohydrate foods each day to meet your child's needs for lunch, snacks, sports, and unexpected extras. It's a good idea to consult with a registered dietitian periodically since your child's energy needs change over time.

THE LOW-GI LUNCH BOX

When it comes to packing your child's lunch, let your imagination be your guide! Try these ideas for starters:

BREAD	+FRUIT	+DAIRY	+DRINK	+SNACKS
Be adventurous with bread choices. Include different bread varieties, rolls, crispbreads, crackers, and muffins.	Include fresh fruit in season—whole, chopped, diced, and sliced. Also serve unsweetened canned fruit packs (in natural juice) and dried fruits.	Include milk (plain or flavored), yogurt (natural, vanilla, or flavored), and cheese.	You can vary drink choices daily. They can include milk, water, flavored seltzers, or fruit juices on occasion. Freeze drinks in summer and store in your child's lunch box to keep the contents cool.	Check the list on page 105 for a wide variety of nourishing, healthy snacks to include in your child's lunch box.

HYPOGLYCEMIA AT SCHOOL

Hypoglycemia can occur at school, so make sure that your child is prepared: In fact, it's a good idea to put together a "low blood-sugar box" for school, which should include some of her favorite high- and low-GI non-perishable finger foods, such as jellybeans, gummy bears, Fruit Roll-ups™, fruit drinks, snack packs of Oreos, Fig Newtons, Lorna Doones, and granola bars.

It's a good idea to leave a couple of these low sugar boxes in strategic locations (one in the classroom, another in the nurse's or principal's office) along with a card that clearly describes the appropriate treatment for your child's hypoglycemia. Be sure to replenish the supplies regularly and check that the foods you pack have not passed their "use-by" date.

If your child appears to have low blood-sugar episodes at school more often than at home, you may want to test her blood at school to confirm whether she's really hypoglycemic. If she is, her doctor may want to change her insulin dose or reassess her diet to make sure that she's getting enough food.

> ### Preventing Late-Morning Hypoglycemia
>
> A common problem for many school children is a delayed recess, which can be as late as 11:00 A.M. Often this gap between breakfast and morning snack is too long, causing hypoglycemia. Some children try to eat during class to prevent hypoglycemia, but this singles them out and may make them feel uncomfortable. Other kids have a small low-GI snack on their way to school, such as dried fruit, flavored milk, a small container of yogurt, whole grain crackers with cheese spread, or peanut butter and all-fruit jelly to keep their blood sugar stable.

Try to include a minimum of one low-GI food per meal and snack per day to achieve good long-term diabetes control.

26

TEENAGERS

THE TEENAGE YEARS tend to be a time when kids want to challenge the world. And some of these challenges include smoking, drinking, skipping insulin (if used), missing meals, and eating whatever! This section provides information that will help parents and teens make good decisions—decisions that will help teens maintain long-term diabetes control and good health.

THE "HOLLOW LEG" SYNDROME

Teenagers tend to grow fast and as a result, are often hungry much of the time. Here's how teens can be more flexible with their diets:

- When they're hungry, teenagers should eat low-GI foods for maximum fill-up value. Good

choices include wholegrain bread, apples, yogurt, pasta, and oatmeal cookies.
- When teens aren't so interested in eating, they can have high-GI foods in smaller amounts, foods such as white bread, cookies, corn flakes, and rice cakes.

TAKE-OUT FOODS

The problem with take-out foods is that kids usually eat them at irregular times and eat greater amounts of sugary or fatty foods than they should as part of a well-balanced low-GI diet. Eating additional carbohydrate food will increase blood-sugar levels.

But, kids don't have to be different. Incorporating low-GI foods whenever possible will let teens enjoy take-out foods without compromising their diabetes control; in fact, as long as they keep some pointers in mind, teens can make fairly healthy food choices at take-out restaurants. Hint: Take-out foods that also happen to have low-GI values include fruit smoothies, ice cream, yogurt, sourdough pretzel nuggets and some types of fresh fruit. Your kids should also:

- choose bottled water, flavored milk, or diet decaffeinated soft drinks rather than regular soft drinks;
- combine any high-GI carbohydrates or saturated fat with low-GI foods; and
- be prepared by having only a light snack after school so they can have an extra snack with their friends.

TYPE OF TAKE-OUT FOOD	BEST CHOICES	FOODS TO LIMIT
McDonald's, Burger King, or other hamburger outlets	Chunky chicken salad Small hamburger Chef salad (use low-fat or fat-free dressing) Chicken tenders Plain ice cream cone Fruit	Deep-fried food Double meat Extra cheese Fried onion rings French fries Bacon Thick shakes Soft drinks
Pizza (takeout/delivery), Chinese take-out	Vegetarian topping Simple cheese topping Braised meat or chicken with steamed rice Stir-fry vegetables or noodles	Pepperoni Double cheese topping Deep-fried egg or spring rolls or dim sum
Sandwich shops, delis, diners	Whole-grain roll or sandwich bread Veggie burger Grilled chicken salad or pita Milkshakes Frozen yogurt Ice cream or frozen yogurt	Pies Sausage rolls French fries Potato chips
Mexican restaurants, such as Taco Bell	Bean burrito Chicken fajita Soft taco Beef taco Tostada with red sauce Frijoles and cheese	Nachos Crispy taco salads Refried beans Guacamole

DRINKING ALCOHOL AND STAYING OUT LATE

Teenagers with diabetes act much like their non-diabetic friends—they may stay out late, sleep in, or drink alcohol. They should talk to their doctor, diabetes educator, or dietitian for advice on how best to deal with all of these situations.

HOW DOES ALCOHOL AFFECT BLOOD-SUGAR LEVELS?

Some drinks, such as beer, mixed drinks, wine coolers, and liqueurs, may initially cause elevated blood sugar or hyperglycemia. But, in general, the biggest problem that comes from combining alcohol with diabetes is actually *low* blood sugar (hypoglycemia), because alcohol prevents the release of stored sugar from the liver. (The body normally calls on these stores if blood-sugar levels drop too low.) Unfortunately, since hypoglycemic and excess alcohol symptoms are similar, your teen's hypoglycemia may go undetected. Stress to your teen the importance of *not* drinking alcohol. As an emergency precaution, make sure that someone in your child's group of friends knows that alcohol can cause her blood sugar to drop so that the friend can help you treat the hypoglycemia, if necessary.

> **Food for Thought**
>
> **YOUR TEEN SHOULD ALWAYS:**
> - carry extra food wherever she's going, and
> - wear some form of diabetes ID (such as an ID bracelet) in case difficulties arise.

■

To help keep blood-sugar levels stable, your teen should be educated on the dangers of alcohol consumption for diabetics.

■

ALCOHOL AND INSULIN

Drinking on an empty stomach leads to higher blood-alcohol levels and, as a result, a greater risk of hypoglycemia. So before your teen with Type 1 diabetes goes out for the night, she should inject her insulin and eat a normal-size low-GI meal—pasta is perfect. She may need to consider lowering her insulin dose, however, if she's lined up lots of activity. She may also need to alter the timing of her doses. (Physical activity tends to lower blood sugar levels.) It would be a good idea for your teen to talk to her diabetes educator to work out an insulin regimen for when she goes out.

WEIGHTY MATTERS

Sometimes the pressures of having a beautiful body seem to clash with the diabetes pressures of eating regularly, eating after exercise, and treating low blood sugars. The good news is, teenagers can maintain a reasonable body weight *and* still control their diabetes.

Becoming overweight is largely an imbalance between activity levels and food intake. If your child honestly thinks she has a weight problem, is worried about how she looks, and wants to diet, she should talk to someone about it; the best choices would be a health professional such as her dietitian, doctor, or diabetes educator. They can help her plan healthy and effective weight management strategies.

DIETARY DON'TS (THEY *DON'T* WORK!)

No matter how good "quick-fix" diets may sound to teenagers, they can all be detrimental to their health. Here are some rules for kids to follow, and the "whys" to back them up. **Don't**:

- **Eliminate** a major food group, such as meat, dairy foods, or starches in the belief that they're fattening foods. The result is a nutritionally inadequate diet with detrimental long-term consequences.
- **Try** a severe low-calorie diet either, because it can dramatically affect your growth and development—and that includes your brain. It's also counterproductive to long-term weight control and will likely bring on a low blood sugar episode.
- **Reduce,** or worse still, skip insulin (if used) in an effort to lose weight. This only results in poor diabetes control. Major adjustments to

your insulin dose (if you use it) or diet are best made under professional guidance.
- **Starve** yourself or go on eating binges followed by purging. If you find yourself doing this, talk to a health professional about it—you could have an eating disorder.
- **Be** tempted to skip meals or snacks in an attempt to reduce the amount of food that you're eating. Skipping meals and snacks not only upsets diabetes control and causes low blood sugar, but also can leave you feeling very hungry and craving junk foods.

JUGGLING SPORTS COMMITMENTS

Playing sports can provide enormous benefits to diabetes control and feelings of well-being. To perform at their best, kids need to monitor the effect that playing a particular sport has on their diabetes control, pay attention to their diet, and plan ahead. They should remember to:

- eat extra carbohydrate during periods of strenuous activity;
- exercise when levels of insulin are not peaking (although this isn't always practical); and
- inject insulin (if used) into an area that is not involved with the vigorous activity.

To deal with before-breakfast training sessions, athletes with diabetes should consume extra low-GI carbohydrate (such as a bowl of old fashioned oats cooked with milk) before training. After finishing training, they should take their insulin dose, if any, then have a normal breakfast around the usual time.

To cope with training/competition during meal and snack times, athletes should eat carbohydrates appropriate for their activity levels, with some additional carbohydrates to allow for any mealtime delays. A combination of low- and high-GI foods would be best.

When teens know they need additional carbohydrate before competing but have no appetite or desire to eat, they should choose light foods or fluids that sit well in their stomachs, such as fruit smoothies, fruit salads, or yogurt.

WORKING PART-TIME

Teens who work part-time may need to alter their usual medication and meal routine to fit in with their scheduled work breaks or negotiate adequate breaks with their employer.

Before starting work, teenagers should have a substantial low-GI meal or snack to help sustain blood-sugar levels. It may be a good idea for kids to take extra carbohydrate snacks such as dried fruits, cookies, granola bars, and fresh fruit from home so that they can eat them on the run. Sometimes small frequent snacks may need to take the place of a full meal break. If the job is quite busy, teens should make sure that they're prepared with extra high-GI carbohydrate snacks; she may want to discuss reducing her insulin dose with her doctor.

◀ 27 ▶

THE FOOD PYRAMID FOR ADOLESCENTS AND TEENAGERS

*I*N ORDER TO grow and develop properly, an adolescent's diet should follow the food groups of the Food Guide Pyramid that appears on page 30. The recommended caloric level for an adolescent should take into account the child's age, gender, current weight status versus ideal or reasonable body weight*, level of physical activity, and growth pattern.

RECOMMENDED FOOD PYRAMID SERVINGS FOR TEENAGERS

As we mentioned earlier, a healthy diet should include low-GI choices from each of the carbohydrate groups below.

FOOD GROUP	SERVINGS FOR TEEN GIRLS	SERVINGS FOR TEEN BOYS
Bread and cereal	9	11
Vegetable	4	5
Fruit	3	4
Milk	3	3
Meat	2 (total 5 ozs.)	3 (total 8 ozs.)

Discourage your kids from consuming too many caffeine-containing foods, including colas, tea, coffee, and chocolate.

DAILY NUTRIENT REQUIREMENTS

Here are some guidelines to help you determine how much your child should be eating.

Calories
Boys
 11–14 years: 41 calories/inch
 15–18 years: 43 calories/inch
Girls
 11–14 years: 36 calories/inch
 15–18 years: 34 calories/inch

Protein
 Approximately 0.4 to 0.5 grams per pound, or 12 to 16 percent of daily calorie intake

Fat

No more than 30 percent of total calories from fat and 10 percent or less of total fat calories from saturated fat

Less than 300 milligrams (mg.) of cholesterol

Calcium

1200 to 1500 mg.

Dietary fiber

5 grams plus child's age (Example: A 15-year-old adolescent should get 5 + 15 = 20 grams of fiber each day.)

*Body Mass Index (BMI) categories to identify adolescents at risk of obesity:

Overweight: BMI 25 to 29.9

At risk: BMI > 30

Calculate Your Body Mass Index (BMI)

TO CALCULATE YOUR BMI, divide your weight (in kilograms) by your height (in meters) squared. To simplify the process, go to http://www.cdc.gov/nccdphp/dnpa/bmi/calc-bmi.htm#English) for an online calculator.

Discourage your kids from eating too much fat, sodium and sugar. These "empty calorie" foods, quite common in teenagers' diets, can easily squeeze out room for healthier food choices.

PART 5

THE GLYCEMIC INDEX MENU PLANNER FOR CHILDREN AND TEENS

◀ 28 ▶

BREAKFAST

*B*REAKFAST IS THE meal that starts the day. It's a great opportunity to optimize your child's use of low-GI foods because so many breakfast foods—breads, cereals, fresh fruits, and dairy foods—are excellent low-GI food sources. Studies have shown that children who eat a nutritious breakfast will perform better, both physically and mentally, than their hungry peers. A wholesome, nutritious, low-GI breakfast ensures optimal performance until the scheduled morning snack. Just make sure that your kids have enough time to enjoy their breakfast without feeling rushed.

Though breakfast is important, many children don't have large appetites at breakfasttime. For small appetites, fruit smoothies and hot chocolate are good starters that will sustain energy levels throughout the morning. Here are some other ideas:

1. **Start with some fruit.**
   Fruit contributes fiber and vitamin C, which helps the body absorb iron.

2. **Try some breakfast cereal.**
   Cereals are important as a source of fiber, vitamin B and iron. When choosing processed breakfast cereals, look for those with a high fiber content (five or more grams per serving). The top four low-GI cereals for children are: old-fashioned oats, granola, Life, and Special K.

3. **Add milk or yogurt.**
   Fat free or low fat milk can make a valuable contribution to your child's daily calcium intake when you include them at breakfast. Both have low-GI values, and low-fat milk varieties have just as much, or more, calcium as whole milk.

4. **Serve some bread or toast.**
   The lowest GI breads are: whole grain pumpernickel rye (GI: 41); sourdough rye (GI: 48); 100% stoneground whole wheat (GI: 53); and whole wheat pita (GI: 57).

FOR TODDLERS

1. Oatmeal and milk and a small glass of apple juice
2. A fruit smoothie—strawberries or peach with milk, yogurt, and honey
3. A small yogurt with fresh fruit salad
4. Scrambled eggs on toast with a small cup of milk
5. Graham crackers with peanut butter and all-fruit jelly

6. Cinnamon toast with a cup of milk
7. "Silver dollar" pancakes and milk

FOR SCHOOL-AGE CHILDREN

1. French toast, made by lightly soaking thick slices of low-GI bread in beaten egg and milk. Sprinkle with cinnamon sugar.
2. A bowl of Just Right with sliced canned peaches and low fat milk
3. Sliced strawberries topped with vanilla yogurt and a sprinkle of Bran Buds or granola
4. Peanut butter and all-fruit jelly on low-GI toast
5. Boiled egg, low-GI toast, and a glass of milk
6. Sourdough English muffin topped with cream cheese

FOR TEENAGERS

1. Bagels
2. Bran, corn, or blueberry muffin with all-fruit jelly
3. French toast with fresh fruit
4. Fruit smoothie
5. Grilled cheese on wholegrain bread
6. Grilled tomato and cheese on toast/muffins
7. Low-GI breakfast cereal with milk and fruit
8. Poached eggs on toast
9. Old-fashioned oats cooked in low fat milk, topped with sliced peaches or cinnamon applesauce
10. Wholegrain toast with peanut butter, or ham and cheese, or eggs
11. Yogurt and fresh fruit and low fat granola

◀ 29 ▶

LUNCHES AND SANDWICH FILLERS

THERE'S NO NEED for children to regard sandwiches with disdain as long as you keep the fillers tasty and creative. Here are some ideas to get you started:

1. Bacon, lettuce, and tomato
2. Egg salad
3. Grilled cheese and tomato
4. Ham, cheese, and salsa
5. Hummus and tomato
6. Lean roast beef and light mayonnaise
7. Mozzarella, roasted peppers, and arugula
8. Peanut butter and all-fruit jelly
9. Tuna salad
10. Veggie burger

SOME TASTY COMBINATIONS

Looking for some food choices that go particularly well together? Try these combos:

Pita pocket filled with tuna salad, diced tomato, and lettuce
Fruit muffin
Small apple and milk
Chicken drumstick with cucumber sticks, cherry tomatoes, and rye crackers
Fruit yogurt
Oatmeal cookies

Soft tortilla filled with ham, cheese, or turkey with diced tomato, pepper, and cucumber
Small container of fresh melon chunks
Frozen flavored milk drink

Roast beef on rye bread with pickle
Container of fruit yogurt
Small container of trail mix

Tossed salad with hard boiled eggs, cheese, olives, and chickpeas
Frozen fruit juice
Container of citrus sections

Food for Thought

- Use different types of bread for variety: Some examples include wholegrain, semolina, sourdough, rye, raisin, muffins, pita, mountain bread, herb bread, and soft tortillas.
- Try to make low-GI sandwiches to help lower the glycemic index for the day.
- Toast sandwiches (such as grilled cheese) the night before; children can eat them cold for lunch the next day for something a little different.

◀ 30 ▶

MAIN MEALS FOR CHILDREN AND TEENS

ONCE YOU KNOW where to start, it's easy to make your child's meals interesting and tasty. Here are some ideas to help get the creativity ball rolling:

FOR TODDLERS

1. Grilled cheese on wholegrain toast (cut into triangles) and a sliced apple
2. Light cream cheese and all-fruit jelly on a sourdough English muffin
3. Macaroni and cheese
4. Tomato soup and low-GI toast

5. Tuna chow mein—canned tuna with fine noodles, stir-fried vegetables, seasoned with soy sauce
6. Vegetable soup with noodles

FOR OLDER CHILDREN AND TEENS

1. Bake a tuna and rice casserole using Uncle Ben's converted or brown rice, peas, corn, and strips of red pepper, topped with ½ cup of light cheese sauce made with skim or reduced fat milk.
2. Bake Tex Mex potatoes (sweet potato baked with onion, bacon, taco seasoning, baked beans, grated cheese, sour cream, and corn chips).
3. Buy a barbecued chicken, steam corn on the cob, and serve with a tossed salad.
4. Buy one or two Chinese take-out stir-fry meals and split them with your family, padding them out with home-cooked low-GI rice or pasta, plus loads of vegetables.
5. Cook a casserole using a good-quality chicken stock and chunks of your child's favorite vegetables, including sweet potato. Serve with brown rice or noodles.
6. Cook spinach and ricotta tortellini, team up with fresh garden vegetables, and top with a tomato sauce.
7. Create a one-pot chicken casserole with your favorite vegetables and chunks of baby new potatoes.
8. Enjoy a risotto made with a low-GI rice, lean meat, fish, or chicken and a variety of vegetables.
9. Grill a steak and serve with a trio of low-GI vegetables—sweet potato, corn, and peas.

10. Grill or barbecue steak (or chicken or fish), serve with a variety of low-GI vegetables (sweet potato, corn, and peas), and crusty whole grain rolls.
11. Make a lasagna—beef and cheese or vegetarian—and serve it with a crispy green salad with lettuce and celery and colorful pepper strips.
12. Serve chili beans and beef with a soft tortilla bread or tacos and a salad.
13. Serve grilled or barbecued sausages and mashed potatoes made with a fifty–fifty mixture of new potato and sweet potato and served with corn on the cob.
14. Serve your favorite pasta (al dente) with a meat sauce or vegetable salsa, and couple it with lightly steamed green vegetables.
15. Stir-fry beef, chicken, or fish and serve with Basmati rice or noodles.
16. Stir-fry chicken, meat, or fish with mixed green vegetables. Serve with brown rice or Chinese noodles.
17. Team spaghetti bolognese with a green salad.
18. Try a corn and green pea frittata, made with eggs and fresh vegetables or a can of corn and a small packet of frozen peas.
19. Wrap a fish fillet dressed with herbs and lemon, or tomato and onion, in foil and bake. Serve with a heavy grain bread roll and salad.

OTHER MEAL IDEAS

1. Make vegetable parcels by combining chopped cooked broccoli, grated carrot, chopped shallots, and sweet corn with ricotta cheese and grated cheddar. Wrap in phyllo pastry and bake until golden.
2. Scoop commercial pasta sauce on pasta with a sprinkle of Parmesan cheese. Add mushrooms, peppers, and other vegetables to the sauce to boost the nutrient value.
3. Serve a casserole with chunky vegetables and sweet potato cubes served with Basmati rice or elbow macaroni.
4. Thread cubes of chicken, beef, or fish onto skewers with button mushrooms, onions, and peppers for a kebab.
5. Microwave a potato and top with broccoli and cheddar cheese.
6. Microwave a veggie burger.
7. Serve nachos or tacos with beef and bean topping, avocado, shredded lettuce, tomato, and reduced-fat grated cheddar cheese.
8. Savor a lentil or split pea soup.

31

JUST DESSERTS

CHILDREN LOVE DESSERTS, which can add calcium and vitamin C to their meals if they're based on low-fat dairy foods and fruits. Recipes incorporating fruit for sweetness will have more fiber and lower GI values than recipes with sugar. What's more, desserts are usually carbohydrate rich, which means they help children feel more full, and reduce the tendency for late night nibbles.

If you don't have time to prepare a dessert, try serving a bowl of in-season fruit or a fruit platter with cheese or yogurt. Remember, temperate climate fruits such as apples, pears, peaches, citrus, and berries tend to have the lowest GI values.

For any of the following suggestions, you should substitute whole milk or whole milk products for children under two years old unless otherwise advised.

QUICK AND EASY LOW-GI DESSERTS

Most everyone looks forward to a sweet, tasty dessert to top off a meal. Here are some simple ideas to end your child's meal in grand style:

1. Combine low-fat ice cream and strawberries.
2. Bake apples whole, and stuff them with dried fruit or tapioca pudding.
3. Enjoy a fruit salad topped with low-fat yogurt.
4. Make a fruit crisp: Top cooked fruit with a crumble mixture of oats, a little melted margarine (poly- or monounsaturated) and honey.
5. Slice a firm banana into some low-fat custard.
6. Top canned fruit (peaches or pears) with low-fat ice cream, low-fat custard, or pudding.
7. Wrap sliced apple, raisins, nuts, and cinnamon in a sheet of phyllo pastry (brushed with milk, not fat) and bake as a strudel.
8. Make a winter fruit salad with segments of citrus fruits and raisins soaked in orange juice and honey.
9. Stew peaches or nectarines and serve them with low-fat frozen yogurt.
10. Make a pudding cooked in low-fat milk.
11. Enjoy a small dish of frozen yogurt.

32

LOW-GI SNACKS

*L*ow-GI foods, as part of your children's meals and snacks, not only help to prevent low blood sugar, but also provide the long-term energy your young ones need to make it through a busy day. Consider these tasty choices:

FOR TODDLERS

1. Blueberry or applesauce muffin
2. Cup of milk and an oatmeal cookie
3. Frozen yogurt
4. Fruit yogurt
5. Raisin toast spread lightly with low-fat cream cheese
6. Slice of fresh low-GI bread with margarine and all-fruit jelly
7. Sliced apple
8. Small bowl of dried fruit—apricot halves, dried apples, and berries

FOR SCHOOL-AGE CHILDREN

1. Canned fruit snack pack
2. Carrot, celery, and zucchini sticks with peanut butter dip
3. Cheese melted on low-GI toast
4. Frozen yogurt on a stick
5. Granola bar
6. Fruit plate of sliced apple, orange rings, grapes, or melon chunks
7. Ice cream cone
8. Tangerines or a bunch of grapes
9. Mini corn cob
10. Corn muffin
11. Vegetable soup with a crusty wholegrain roll
12. Yogurt with Grape-Nuts or low fat granola

FOR TEENAGERS

1. Apple or pear
2. Muffins or raisin bread
3. Leftovers—pizza, rice, noodles
4. Low-fat ice cream
5. Low-fat milk
6. Nachos—corn chips and melted cheese
7. Nutri-Grain bars
8. Pasta snack
9. Smoothie
10. Grilled sandwich made with low-GI bread

33

PARTY IDEAS

*Y*OUR CHILD SHOULDN'T miss out on party fun and fare just because she has diabetes. Within reason, relax her diet for that special meal or snack and allow a moderate number of party treats. Having one slice of birthday cake is sensible, for example, but going back for a third helping is not. Encourage her to bring home the goodie bag, which she can have either as dessert that evening or before exercise later. An occasional rise in blood-sugar level on special occasions does no harm. It's what you do the remainder of the time that is more important.

On the day of the party, keep the insulin dose (if any) the same (even though it is likely that she'll eat extra). Remember that she may be more active at the party, which would allow her to eat the extra party food without increasing her blood-sugar levels too dramatically.

If her blood sugar is high after the party, don't panic. Make sure she eats her dinner and bedtime snack so that her blood-sugar levels don't drop rapidly overnight.

> **Many parents are surprised at how good their child's blood-sugar readings are after parties.**

PARTY FARE

When children go to parties, what they eat depends largely on what the hosts offer. If you know the party hosts, you can call them ahead of time to find out what they're serving. If that's not an option for you, you could have your child bring a tasty treat for all the guests to share.

Here are some ideas of foods you could bring, or serve when the party is at your house:

Cakes, cookies, ice cream (made with artificial sweeteners, alternative sweeteners such as fructose, fruit juice, or fruit purees, or reduced amounts of sugar)
Calzones
Chicken nuggets
Chili
Chips and salsa
Decaf diet beverages
Lasagna
Nuts
Sloppy Joe pitas
Spaghetti and meatballs
Sweet potato fries
Tacos
Tortilla wraps
Veggies and dips
White pizza

34

OTHER LOW-GI DIETS

A LOW-GI DIET AND CELIAC DISEASE

*A*pproximately **1** in 20 people with diabetes also suffer from celiac disease, an autoimmune disorder in which the protein, gluten, causes a reaction that damages the lining of the small intestine. As a result, people with celiac disease need to follow a gluten-free diet for the rest of their lives. Gluten is found in products made from wheat, rye, and barley and in foods such as breads, pasta, and cookies. Luckily, there are many gluten-free products available on the market to replace these staple foods. It can sometimes be tricky trying to follow a low-GI diet on a gluten-free diet, though, since many popular low-GI foods also contain gluten.

Here are two easy ways to help manage a low-GI, gluten-free diet:

- Make the most of naturally gluten-free, low-GI foods, such as fruits, vegetables, legumes, and most dairy foods.
- Try sweet potatoes, baked beans, corn, brown or Basmati rice, kidney beans, lentils, or chickpeas in main meals as low-GI, gluten-free alternatives to potato.

Try some of the following foods for a low-GI, gluten-free snack:

- Fresh fruit
- Ice cream
- Nuts (for children older than age five)
- Corn chips and dip
- Yogurt (check ingredients)
- Smoothie or milkshake
- Plain potato chips
- Canned fruit
- Dried apples, apricots, or raisins

Menu suggestions for celiac disease and diabetes

Breakfast:
Gluten-free breakfast cereal and milk.
Toast (gluten-free bread)
Gluten-free pancakes
Fresh or canned fruit in natural juice
Milk

Lunch:
Sandwich (gluten-free bread)
Cold chicken or roast meat and salad (include sweet potato or a rice salad for carbohydrate)
Yogurt (check ingredients)
Fresh fruit or fruit snack packs
Dried fruit and nuts

Afternoon snack:
Select from snack list on page 105.

Dinner:
Plain meat without a sauce, unless it's gluten-free
Gluten-free pasta, low-GI rice, and legumes
Stir-fry with gluten-free noodles or rice
Canned or fresh fruit with ice cream or yogurt (check ingredients)

Evening snack:
Select from snack list on page 105.

A LOW-GI DIET AND INSULIN PUMPS

Some young people with diabetes are now being treated with insulin pump therapy. An insulin pump administers a continuous insulin infusion throughout the day, with extra insulin given as a bolus dose at meal/snack times. The aim of pump therapy is to achieve very tight blood glucose control, because the pump gives you the ability to finely adjust your child's insulin needs depending on their food intake, activity, and blood-glucose level.

From our knowledge of the glycemic index, we know

that different carbohydrate foods affect the blood-glucose level differently. With intense pre-meal and post-meal blood glucose monitoring it becomes obvious that some carbohydrate foods or particular meals cause a higher after-meal blood-glucose level than others. Insulin pump therapy allows you to adapt not only your child's bolus insulin dose but also the bolus type (such as normal bolus, dual-wave bolus or square-wave bolus options) to better suit your child's blood-glucose profile.

Knowledge of the glycemic values of particular foods or the glycemic load of particular meal combinations becomes even more important in managing your child's diabetes because this knowledge will help you predict the type of bolus and amount of insulin necessary to achieve ideal blood-glucose control.

PART 6

YOUR QUESTIONS ANSWERED

35

THE MEAL SKIPPERS

My daughter refuses to eat breakfast and I'm worried that she will become hypoglycemic on the way to school. What should I do?

Breakfast is an important meal to start the day and skipping this meal should not be an option for any child with diabetes. Breakfast provides you with a great opportunity to include plenty of low-GI foods because many breakfast items—breads, cereals, fresh fruits and dairy foods—have low-GI values. Some children don't have large appetites at breakfast time, so it is important to optimize carbohydrate intake.

Make sure there is plenty of time to enjoy a good breakfast. Milkshakes, fruit smoothies, and hot chocolate are good starters. All of these foods have low-GI values that will sustain blood-sugar levels for longer periods. And negotiate foods that she will eat—they needn't necessarily be traditional breakfast foods.

Check the low-GI breakfast list on page 94 for some creative ideas.

She may prefer two small low-GI snacks (one at breakfast and one on the way to school), which will ensure that she gets enough carbohydrate to minimize the risk of low blood sugar.

When my son is invited to parties he gets so busy playing that he hardly eats and always ends up hypoglycemic. What should I do?

Give your son a low-GI snack before he goes to the party so that what he eats once he gets there will not be as important. Low-GI snacks will help him maintain blood-sugar control and will lessen the blood-sugar effects of any party foods he does eat.

My son eats too much after school, then has high blood-sugar readings and is never hungry at dinnertime. What should I do?

Your son is hungry and eating large quantities of food in the afternoon when the effects of his long-acting insulin are wearing off; that's why his blood-sugar level is elevated.

First, watch the foods he eats for his afternoon snack. High-fat snack foods, such as chips or sweet cookies, don't satisfy an appetite. Try combining these foods with some low-GI choices (such as fruit, sandwiches made with wholegrain breads or rolls, or milk) that will satisfy his appetite and have a minimal impact on his blood sugar.

Try to understand why he's so hungry. Is he eating enough during the day? Providing low-GI food choices for him to eat throughout the day, particularly his school lunch, may help alleviate that ravenous after-school appetite.

Is he eating because he's bored? Suggest that once he's had his snack he get away from food and get busy.

Alternatively, maybe his insulin regime can be adjusted. He might try dividing his pre-dinner insulin dose into two separate injections by giving himself the short-acting insulin after school. That way he'll have adequate insulin to cope with his large after-school appetite. He may then take his long-acting insulin before supper. Effectively, he'll be giving himself three injections of insulin per day so that the peak action of insulin is better matched to his food intake and blood-sugar profile. Discuss these options with your son's diabetes care team.

NO SPECIAL TREATS REQUIRED

I spend weekends baking special sugar-free cakes and cookies for my son's school lunch to try to give him more variety, but these foods always come home uneaten. Can you suggest any special recipe books?

There's no need to use special sugar-free recipes or artificial sweeteners: Using moderate amounts of sugar in cooking is fine and won't interfere with your son's diabetes control as long as you count these foods as part of his total carbohydrate intake. Bake your family's favorite recipes, and remember that it's more likely that you'll need to reduce the fat content of your recipes than the sugar content.

CANDY CONCERNS

My child, who takes insulin, is very active during playtime at school so I pack candy in his lunch box every day to prevent low blood sugar. Now he eats more candy than he ever did before he was diagnosed with diabetes. Does this seem right?

Your child should not need candy every day to prevent dips in blood sugar. Even if he is very active at play, his regular insulin dose and food intake should be appropriate for his activity level. Additional carbohydrate foods are only required for extra strenuous activity. If you find that your child needs to eat extra food regularly, discuss his current insulin regimen with his doctor and have a registered dietitian review his calorie intake.

HYPOGLYCEMIA AFTER SPORTS

My type 1 son is very active and attends track practice three afternoons a week. He always eats extra foods before training but seems to experience hypoglycemia in the late evening after each session. Is there something more he should be doing?

Delayed hypoglycemia after strenuous activity is usually an indication that your son requires either more carbohydrate or less insulin. During the activity he may have used the glucose stored in his liver, and it isn't until later in the evening, when his body tries to replenish its stores, that the hypoglycemia occurs. He can prevent this from happening by eating some high-GI carbohydrate prior to, during or immediately after the event. Alternatively, he could reduce his insulin dose if he doesn't want to eat more carbohydrate. He should make sure that his dinner and bedtime snack contain additional low-GI carbohydrate foods to sustain his blood-sugar levels overnight.

Appetite is often a good guide to help determine whether your son needs additional carbohydrate. We recommend that he eat extra low-GI foods at dinner and/or bedtime to match his appetite after very strenuous activities. It may be a good idea for your son to check his blood-sugar levels more frequently—at least temporarily—before, during, immediately following and approximately four to six hours after his training sessions. The results will provide him with valuable blood-sugar information so that he can make better decisions regarding any insulin/food changes.

INFANT AND TODDLER CONCERNS

How can I tell if my breast-fed baby is getting enough breast milk to avoid hypoglycemia?

If your baby is thriving, gaining the appropriate amount of weight, has an adequate number of wet diapers, appears settled after feedings, and is demand feeding every two to three hours throughout the day, the chances are that your baby is receiving enough and doing well. You can also regularly monitor her blood-sugar level to reassure yourself that you're meeting her needs.

Should I introduce solids to my baby before she's five months old?

No. There is no benefit in introducing solids before

five months of age. A baby's digestive system is still immature and not ready to cope with solid foods before then. Introducing foods earlier may increase your baby's chances of developing food allergies and diarrhea (due to undigested food); it can also lead to poor growth. If you think your baby is hungry, offer more breast milk or formula feedings until she's ready to start solids.

What is the best way to manage low blood sugars in an infant?

Treat hypoglycemia by giving your infant glucose syrup either from a plastic eye dropper or a soft plastic spoon, followed by a breast- or formula feeding as soon as possible.

My toddler is so tired by the end of the day, he won't eat his evening meal and I am frightened that his blood sugar will drop in the middle of the night. What should I do?

It isn't unusual for tired toddlers to be uninterested in the evening meal; in fact, they can often be quite distracted if the whole family is sitting down together. Feeding your toddler earlier in the evening (5:00 or 5:30 P.M.) before fatigue sets in may help. Then they can sit with the family at the later mealtime without the pressure. If they consume more food during your family's evening meal, it's a bonus.

Another approach would be to give toddlers their main meal at lunchtime when their appetites may be better. You can then offer a lighter evening meal, such as sandwiches, fruit or yogurt. Check the meal and snack suggestions on pages 99 and 105 for ways to incorporate low-GI foods into your child's usual food choices. A bottle or cup of milk before bed is a common routine in this age group and may help to satisfy their appetite for a longer period since low-GI foods (such as milk) make them feel fuller longer. It also can be helpful and reassuring to monitor your child's blood sugar at bedtime.

My two-year-old girl's blood sugars are never stable. How can I determine what I'm doing wrong?

Be reassured that you are not the only parent of a toddler with diabetes who is frustrated with unstable diabetes control. We don't aim for tight control because detecting and treating low blood sugar in this age group is a difficult task, because toddlers are too young to recognize the symptoms. Experts accept a wider blood-sugar range in this age group because kids' activity levels are erratic and their food intake can be unpredictable. Your child's HbA1c results are often a better indication of their overall diabetes control than the highly fluctuating daily blood tests. (Hemoglobin A1c is a blood test that gives a person's blood-sugar average for the prior two to three months.)

Incorporating low-GI foods over the course of the day may help to minimize the rapid blood sugar fluctuations, but it certainly won't prevent them. If you can manage your toddler's diabetes so that she is free of hypoglycemia and ketones, you're doing a fabulous job.

My two-year-old son is about to start childcare. How can I be sure that his diabetes will be managed properly?

One of the hardest things about being a parent is letting

go as your toddler becomes more independent and others assume responsibility for his well-being. You need to feel confident that the staff is able to manage his diabetes: They need to be made aware of his usual routines and know how to recognize and treat symptoms of hypoglycemia.

In our experience, there have been no difficulties with children attending childcare: The days are structured and the meals they supply are nutritious and appropriate. If you feel that this isn't the case, though, you could send your child's food with him each day. Your diabetes educator may be able to visit the center or provide you with written information to pass on to the staff.

PART 7

THE GI TABLES

36

LET'S TALK GLYCEMIC LOAD

*I*N ADDITION TO the GI values we provide in this book, our tables also include the glycemic load (GL) value for average-sized food portions. Taken together, the glycemic index and glycemic load provide you with all the information you need to choose a diet brimming with health-boosting foods.

GLYCEMIC LOAD 101

A food's glycemic load results from the GI value and carbohydrate per serving of food. When we eat a carbohydrate-containing meal, our blood glucose first rises, then falls. The extent to which it rises and remains high is critically important to our health and depends on two things: the *amount* of a carbohydrate in the meal and the *nature* (GI value) of that carbohydrate. Both factors equally determine blood-glucose changes.

Researchers at Harvard University came up with a way of combining and describing these two factors with the term "glycemic load," which not only provides a measure of the level of glucose in the blood, but also the insulin demand produced by a normal serving of the food. Researchers measure GI values for fixed portions of foods containing a certain amount of carbohydrate (usually 50 grams). Then, as people eat different-sized portions of the same foods, we can work out the extent to which a certain portion of food will raise the blood-glucose level by calculating a glycemic load value for that amount of food.

To calculate glycemic load, multiply a food's GI value by the amount of carbohydrate in a particular serving size, then divide by 100.

Glycemic load = (GI Value x carbohydrate per serving) ÷ 100

For example, a small apple has a GI value of 40 and contains 15 grams of carbohydrate. Its glycemic load is (40 × 15) ÷ 100 = 6. A small 5-ounce potato has a GI value of 90 and 15 grams of carbohydrate. It has a glycemic load of (90 × 15) ÷ 100 = 14. This means one small potato will raise your blood-glucose level higher than one apple.

Low GL = 10 or less
Intermediate GL = 11–19
High GL = 20 or more

> ### How GI Values Affect Glycemic Load
>
> **THE GLYCEMIC LOAD** is greatest for those foods that provide the highest-GI carbohydrate, particularly those we tend to eat in large quantities. Compare the glycemic load of the following foods to see how the serving size, as well as the GI value, help to determine the glycemic response:
>
> | Rice, 1 cup | Spaghetti, 1 cup |
> |---|---|
> | Carbohydrates: 43 | Carbohydrates: 40 |
> | GI: 83 | GI: 44 |
> | GL: 36 | GL: 18 |
> | (83 × 43) ÷ 100 = 36 | (44 × 40) ÷ 100 = 18 |

Some nutritionists argue that the glycemic load is an improvement on the glycemic index because it provides an estimate of both quantity *and* quality of carbohydrate (the GI value gives us just quality) in a diet. In large Harvard studies, however, researchers were able to predict disease risk from people's overall diet, as well as its glycemic load. Using the glycemic load strengthened the relationship, suggesting that the more frequently we consume high-carbohydrate, high-GI foods, the worse it is for our health. Carbohydrate by itself has no effect—in other words, there was no benefit of low-carbohydrate intake over high-carbohydrate intake, or vice versa.

Remember that the GL values we provide are for the standardized (nominal) portion sizes listed. If you eat a different portion size, then you'll need to calculate another GI value. Here's how: First, determine the size of your portion, then work out the available carbohydrate content of this weight (this value is listed next to the GL), then multiply by the food's GI value. For example, the nominal serving size listed for bran flakes is ½ cup, the available carbohydrate is 18 grams, and the GI value is 74. So the GL for ½-cup serving of bran flakes is (74 × 18) ÷ 100 = 13. If, however, you normally eat 1 cup of bran flakes, you'd need to double the available carbohydrate (18 × 2 = 36), and the GL for your larger cereal portion would be (74 × 36) ÷ 100 = 27. These numbers show that the larger portion of cereal releases a larger quantity of glucose into the bloodstream.

We urge you not to make the mistake of using the glycemic load alone. If you do, you might find yourself eating a diet with very little carbohydrate but a lot of fat—especially saturated fat—and excessive amounts of protein. For your overall health, the fat, fiber, and micronutrient content of your diet is also important. A dietitian can guide you further with healthy food choices.

◀ 37 ▶

A TO Z
GI VALUES

THE TABLE IN this section will help you find a food's glycemic index value quickly and easily, because we've listed the foods alphabetically.

The list provides not only the food's GI value but also its glycemic load (GL = (carbohydrate content × GI value) ÷ 100). We calculate the glycemic load using a "nominal" serving size as well as the carbohydrate content of that serving—both of which we've also listed. That way, you can choose foods with either a low-GI value or a low-glycemic load. If your favorite food is both high-GI and high-GL, you can either cut down the serving size or dilute the GL by combining it with very-low-GI foods, such as rice and lentils.

For the first time, we've also included foods that have very little carbohydrate; their GI value is zero, indicated by [0]. Many vegetables, such as avocados and broccoli, and protein foods such as chicken, cheese, and tuna, fall into the low- or no-carbohydrate category. Most alcoholic beverages are also low in carbohydrate.

> **Key to the Table**
>
> **GI Value:** The glycemic index value for the food, where glucose equals 100
>
> **Nominal Serving Size:** The portion of food tested
>
> **Net Carb per Serving:** The total grams of carbs available to the body for digestion from the particular food in the specific serving size (total grams of carbs minus grams of fiber)
>
> **GL per Serving:** Glycemic load of the food; this relates to the quantity of carbs that will enter the bloodstream for the particular food in the specific serving size

POCKET GUIDE TO CHILDHOOD DIABETES

FOOD	GI Value	Nominal Serving Size	Net Carb per Serving	GL per Serving
A				
All-Bran®, breakfast cereal	30	½ cup	15	4
Almonds	[0]	1.75 oz	0	0
Angel food cake, 1 slice	67	1/12 cake	29	19
Apple, dried	29	9 rings	34	10
Apple, fresh, medium	38	4 oz	15	6
Apple juice, pure, unsweetened, reconstituted	40	8 oz	29	12
Apple muffin, small	44	3.5 oz	41	18
Apricots, canned in light syrup	64	4 halves	19	12
Apricots, dried	30	17 halves	27	8
Apricots, fresh, 3 medium	57	4 oz	9	5
Arborio, risotto rice, cooked	69	¾ cup	53	36
Artichokes (Jerusalem)	[0]	½ cup	0	0
Avocado	[0]	¼	0	0
B				
Bagel, white	72	½	35	25
Baked beans	38	⅔ cup	31	12
Baked beans, canned in tomato sauce	48	⅔ cup	15	7
Banana cake, 1 slice	47	⅛ cake	38	18
Banana, fresh, medium	52	4 oz	24	12
Barley, pearled, cooked	25	1 cup	42	11
Basmati rice, white, cooked	58	1 cup	38	22
Beef	[0]	4 oz	0	0
Beer	[0]	8 oz	10	0
Beets, canned	64	½ cup	7	5
Bengal gram dahl, chickpea	11	5 oz	36	4
Black bean soup	64	1 cup	27	17
Black beans, cooked	30	⅘ cup	23	7
Black-eyed peas, canned	42	⅔ cup	17	7

[0] indicates that the food has so little carbohydrate that the GI value cannot be tested. The GL, therefore, is 0.

FOOD	GI Value	Nominal Serving Size	Net Carb per Serving	GL per Serving
Blueberry muffin, small	59	3.5 oz	47	28
Bok choy, raw	[0]	1 cup	0	0
Bran Flakes™, breakfast cereal	74	½ cup	18	13
Bran muffin, small	60	3.5 oz	41	25
Brandy	[0]	1 oz	0	0
Brazil nuts	[0]	1.75 oz	0	0
Breton wheat crackers	67	6 crackers	14	10
Broad beans	79	½ cup	11	9
Broccoli, raw	[0]	1 cup	0	0
Broken rice, white, cooked	86	1 cup	43	37
Brown rice, cooked	50	1 cup	33	16
Buckwheat	54	¾ cup	30	16
Bulgur, cooked 20 min	48	¾ cup	26	12
Bun, hamburger	61	1.5 oz	22	13
Butter beans, canned	31	⅔ cup	20	6

C

FOOD	GI Value	Nominal Serving Size	Net Carb per Serving	GL per Serving
Cabbage, raw	[0]	1 cup	0	0
Cactus Nectar, Organic Agave, light, 90% fructose (Western Commerce)	11	1 Tbsp	8	1
Cactus Nectar, Organic Agave, light, 97% fructose (Western Commerce)	10	1 Tbsp	8	1
Cantaloupe, fresh	65	4 oz	6	4
Cappellini pasta, cooked	45	1½ cups	45	20
Carrot juice, fresh	43	8 oz	23	10
Carrots, peeled, cooked	49	½ cup	5	2
Carrots, raw	47	1 medium	6	3
Cashew nuts, salted	22	1.75 oz	13	3
Cauliflower, raw	[0]	¾ cup	0	0
Celery, raw	[0]	2 stalks	0	0
Cheese	[0]	4 oz	0	0

[0] indicates that the food has so little carbohydrate that the GI value cannot be tested. The GL, therefore, is 0.

POCKET GUIDE TO CHILDHOOD DIABETES 133

FOOD	GI Value	Nominal Serving Size	Net Carb per Serving	GL per Serving
Cherries, fresh	22	18	12	3
Chicken nuggets, frozen	46	4 oz	16	7
Chickpeas, canned	42	⅔ cup	22	9
Chickpeas, dried, cooked	28	⅔ cup	30	8
Chocolate cake made from mix with chocolate frosting	38	4 oz	52	20
Chocolate milk, low-fat	34	8 oz	26	9
Chocolate mousse, 2% fat	31	½ cup	22	7
Chocolate powder, dissolved in water	55	8 oz	16	9
Chocolate pudding, made from powder and whole milk	47	½ cup	24	11
Choice DM™, nutritional support product, vanilla (Mead Johnson)	23	8 oz	24	6
Clif® bar (cookies & cream)	101	2.4 oz	34	34
Coca Cola®, soft drink	53	8 oz	26	14
Cocoa Puffs™, breakfast cereal	77	1 cup	26	20
Complete™, breakfast cereal	48	1 cup	21	10
Condensed milk, sweetened	61	2½ Tbsps	27	17
Converted rice, long-grain, cooked 20-30 min, Uncle Ben's®	50	1 cup	36	18
Converted rice, white, cooked 20-30 min, Uncle Ben's®	38	1 cup	36	14
Corn Flakes™, breakfast cereal	92	1 cup	26	24
Corn Flakes™, Honey Crunch, breakfast cereal	72	¾ cup	25	18
Corn pasta, gluten-free	78	1¼ cups	42	32
Corn Pops™, breakfast cereal	80	1 cup	26	21
Corn Thins, puffed corn cakes, gluten-free	87	1 oz	20	18
Corn, sweet, cooked	60	½ cup	18	11
Cornmeal, cooked 2 min	68	1 cup	13	9
Couscous, cooked 5 min	65	¾ cup	35	23

[0] indicates that the food has so little carbohydrate that the GI value cannot be tested. The GL, therefore, is 0.

134 THE NEW GLUCOSE REVOLUTION

FOOD	GI Value	Nominal Serving Size	Net Carb per Serving	GL per Serving
Cranberry juice cocktail	52	8 oz	31	16
Crispix™, breakfast cereal	87	1 cup	25	22
Croissant, medium	67	2 oz	26	17
Cucumber, raw	[0]	¾ cup	0	0
Cupcake, strawberry-iced, small	73	1.5 oz	26	19
Custard apple, raw, flesh only	54	4 oz	19	10
Custard, homemade	43	½ cup	26	11
Custard, prepared from powder with whole milk, instant	35	½ cup	26	9

D

FOOD	GI Value	Nominal Serving Size	Net Carb per Serving	GL per Serving
Dates, dried	50	7	40	20
Desiree potato, peeled, cooked	101	5 oz	17	17
Doughnut, cake type	76	1.75 oz	23	17

E

FOOD	GI Value	Nominal Serving Size	Net Carb per Serving	GL per Serving
Eggs, large	[0]	2	0	0
Enercal Plus™ (Wyeth-Ayerst)	61	8 oz	40	24
English Muffin™ bread (Natural Ovens)	77	1 oz	14	11
Ensure™, vanilla drink	48	8 oz	34	16
Ensure™ bar, chocolate fudge brownie	43	1.4 oz	20	8
Ensure Plus™, vanilla drink	40	8 oz	47	19
Ensure Pudding™, old-fashioned vanilla	36	4 oz	26	9

F

FOOD	GI Value	Nominal Serving Size	Net Carb per Serving	GL per Serving
Fanta®, orange soft drink	68	8 oz	34	23
Fettuccine, egg, cooked	32	1½ cups	46	15
Figs, dried	61	3	26	16
Fish	[0]	4 oz	0	0
Fish sticks	38	3.5 oz	19	7
Flan/crème caramel	65	½ cup	73	47
French baguette, white, plain	95	1 oz	15	15

[0] indicates that the food has so little carbohydrate that the GI value cannot be tested. The GL, therefore, is 0.

FOOD	GI Value	Nominal Serving Size	Net Carb per Serving	GL per Serving
French fries, frozen, reheated in microwave	75	30 pcs	29	22
French green beans, cooked	[0]	½ cup	0	0
French vanilla cake made from mix, with vanilla frosting	42	4 oz	58	24
French vanilla ice cream, premium, 16% fat	38	½ cup	14	5
Froot Loops™, breakfast cereal	69	1 cup	26	18
Frosted Flakes™, breakfast cereal	55	1 cup	26	15
Fructose, pure	19	1 Tbsp	10	2
Fruit cocktail, canned, light syrup	55	½ cup	16	9
Fruit leather	61	2 pcs	24	15

G

FOOD	GI Value	Nominal Serving Size	Net Carb per Serving	GL per Serving
Gatorade™ (orange) sports drink	89	8 oz	15	13
Gin	[0]	1 oz	0	0
Glucerna™, vanilla (Abbott)	31	8 oz	23	7
Glucose (dextrose)	99	1 Tbsp	10	10
Glucose tablets	102	3 pcs	15	15
Gluten-free corn pasta	78	1½ cups	42	32
Gluten-free multigrain bread	79	1 oz	13	10
Gluten-free rice and corn pasta	76	1½ cups	49	37
Gluten-free spaghetti, rice and split pea, canned in tomato sauce	68	8 oz	27	19
Gluten-free split pea and soy pasta shells	29	1½ cups	31	9
Gluten-free white bread, sliced	80	1 oz	15	12
Glutinous (sticky) rice, white, cooked	92	⅔ cup	48	44
Gnocchi	68	6 oz	48	33
Grapefruit, fresh, medium	25	1 half	11	3
Grapefruit juice, unsweetened	48	8 oz	20	9
Grape-Nuts® (Post), breakfast cereal	75	¼ cup	21	16

[0] indicates that the food has so little carbohydrate that the GI value cannot be tested. The GL, therefore, is 0.

THE NEW GLUCOSE REVOLUTION

FOOD	GI Value	Nominal Serving Size	Net Carb per Serving	GL per Serving
Grapes, black, fresh	59	¾ cup	18	11
Grapes, green, fresh	46	¾ cup	18	8
Green peas	48	½ cup	7	3
Green pea soup, canned	66	8 oz	41	27

H

FOOD	GI Value	Nominal Serving Size	Net Carb per Serving	GL per Serving
Hamburger bun	61	1.5 oz	22	13
Happiness™ (cinnamon, raisin, pecan bread) (Natural Ovens)	63	1 oz	14	9
Hazelnuts	[0]	1.75 oz	0	0
Healthy Choice™ Hearty 100% Whole Grain	62	1 oz	14	9
Healthy Choice™ Hearty 7-Grain	55	1 oz	14	8
Heary Oatmeal cookies, Fifty50	30	4 cookies	20	6
Honey	55	1 Tbsp	18	10
Honey graham crackers	74	9 squares	18 squares	13
Hot cereal, apple & cinnamon, dry (ConAgra)	37	1.2 oz	22	8
Hot cereal, unflavored, dry (ConAgra)	25	1.2 oz	19	5
Hunger Filler™, whole-grain bread (Natural Ovens)	59	1 oz	13	7

I

FOOD	GI Value	Nominal Serving Size	Net Carb per Serving	GL per Serving
Ice cream, low-fat, vanilla, "light"	50	½ cup	9	5
Ice cream, premium, French vanilla, 16% fat	38	½ cup	14	5
Ice cream, premium, "ultra chocolate," 15% fat	37	½ cup	14	5
Ice cream, regular fat	61	½ cup	20	12
Instant potato, mashed	97	¾ cup	20	17
Instant rice, white, cooked 6 min	74	¾ cup	42	36
Ironman PR® bar, chocolate	39	2.3 oz	26	10

[0] indicates that the food has so little carbohydrate that the GI value cannot be tested. The GL, therefore, is 0.

FOOD	GI Value	Nominal Serving Size	Net Carb per Serving	GL per Serving
J				
Jam, apricot fruit spread, reduced sugar	55	1½ Tbsps	13	7
Jam, strawberry	51	1½ Tbsps	20	10
Jasmine rice, white, cooked	109	1 cup	42	46
Jelly beans	78	10 large	28	22
K				
Kaiser roll	73	1 half	16	12
Kavli™ Norwegian crispbread	71	5 pcs	16	12
Kidney beans, canned	52	⅔ cup	17	9
Kidney beans, cooked	23	⅔ cup	25	6
Kiwi fruit	53	4 oz	12	7
Kudos® Whole Grain Bars, chocolate chip	62	1.8 oz	32	20
L				
Lactose, pure	46	1 Tbsp	10	5
Lamb	[0]	4 oz	0	0
Leafy vegetables (spinach, arugula, etc.), raw	[0]	1½ cups	0	0
L.E.A.N Fibergy™ bar, Harvest Oat	45	1.75 oz	29	13
L.E.A.N Life long Nutribar™, Chocolate Crunch	32	1.5 oz	19	6
L.E.A.N Life long Nutribar™, Peanut Crunch	30	1.5 oz	19	6
L.E.A.N Nutrimeal™, drink powder, Dutch Chocolate	26	8 oz	13	3
Lemonade, reconstituted	66	8 oz	20	13
Lentil soup, canned	44	9 oz	21	9
Lentils, brown, cooked	29	¾ cup	18	5
Lentils, green, cooked	30	¾ cup	17	5
Lentils, red, cooked	26	¾ cup	18	5

[0] indicates that the food has so little carbohydrate that the GI value cannot be tested. The GL, therefore, is 0.

THE NEW GLUCOSE REVOLUTION

FOOD	GI Value	Nominal Serving Size	Net Carb per Serving	GL per Serving
Lettuce	[0]	4 leaves	0	0
Life Savers®, peppermint candy	70	18 pcs	30	21
Light rye bread	68	1 oz	14	10
Lima beans, baby, frozen	32	¾ cup	30	10
Linguine pasta, thick, cooked	46	1½ cups	48	22
Linguine pasta, thin, cooked	52	1½ cups	45	23
Long-grain rice, cooked 10 min	61	1 cup	36	22
Lychees, canned in syrup, drained	79	4 oz	20	16

M

FOOD	GI Value	Nominal Serving Size	Net Carb per Serving	GL per Serving
M & M's®, peanut	33	15 pcs	17	6
Macadamia nuts	[0]	1.75 oz	0	0
Macaroni and cheese, made from mix	64	1 cup	51	32
Macaroni, cooked	47	1¼ cups	48	23
Maltose	105	1 Tbsp	10	11
Mango	51	4 oz	15	8
Maple syrup, pure Canadian	54	1 Tbsp	18	10
Marmalade, orange	48	1½ Tbsps	20	9
Mars Bar®	68	2 oz	40	27
Melba toast, Old London	70	6 pcs	23	16
METRx® bar (vanilla)	74	3.6 oz	50	37
Milk Arrowroot™ cookies	69	5	18	12
Millet, cooked	71	⅔ cup	36	25
Mini Wheats™, whole-wheat breakfast cereal	58	12 pcs	21	12
Mousse, butterscotch, 1.9% fat	36	1.75 oz	10	4
Mousse, chocolate, 2% fat	31	1.75 oz	11	3
Mousse, hazelnut, 2.4% fat	36	1.75 oz	10	4
Mousse, mango, 1.8% fat	33	1.75 oz	11	4
Mousse, mixed berry, 2.2% fat	36	1.75 oz	10	4
Mousse, strawberry, 2.3% fat	32	1.75 oz	10	3

[0] indicates that the food has so little carbohydrate that the GI value cannot be tested. The GL, therefore, is 0.

POCKET GUIDE TO CHILDHOOD DIABETES

FOOD	GI Value	Nominal Serving Size	Net Carb per Serving	GL per Serving
Muesli bar containing dried fruit	61	1 oz	21	13
Muesli bread, made from mix in bread oven (ConAgra)	54	1 oz	12	7
Muesli, gluten-free, with low-fat milk	39	1 oz	19	7
Muesli, Swiss Formula	56	1 oz	16	9
Muesli, toasted	43	1 oz	17	7
Multi-Grain 9-Grain bread	43	1 oz	14	6

N

FOOD	GI Value	Nominal Serving Size	Net Carb per Serving	GL per Serving
Navy beans, canned	38	5 oz	31	12
Nesquik™, chocolate dissolved in low-fat milk, no-sugar-added	41	8 oz	11	5
Nesquik™, strawberry dissolved in low-fat milk, no-sugar-added	35	8 oz	12	4
New creamer potato, canned	65	5 oz	18	12
New creamer potato, unpeeled and cooked 20 min	78	5 oz	21	16
Noodles, instant "two-minute" (Maggi®)	46	1½ cups	40	19
Noodles, mung bean (Lungkow beanthread), dried, cooked	39	1½ cups	45	18
Noodles, rice, fresh, cooked	40	1½ cups	39	15
Nutella®, chocolate hazelnut spread	33	1 Tbsp	12	4
Nutrigrain™, breakfast cereal	66	1 cup	15	10
Nutty Natural™, whole-grain bread (Natural Ovens)	59	1 oz	12	7

O

FOOD	GI Value	Nominal Serving Size	Net Carb per Serving	GL per Serving
Oat bran, raw	55	2 Tbsp	5	3
Oatmeal, cooked 1 min	66	1 cup	26	17
Oatmeal cookies	55	4 small	21	12
Oatmeal cookies, Sugar-Free, Fifty50	47	4 cookies	28	10

[0] indicates that the food has so little carbohydrate that the GI value cannot be tested. The GL, therefore, is 0.

THE NEW GLUCOSE REVOLUTION

FOOD	GI Value	Nominal Serving Size	Net Carb per Serving	GL per Serving
Orange juice, unsweetened, reconstituted	53	8 oz	18	9
Orange, fresh, medium	42	4 oz	11	5

P

FOOD	GI Value	Nominal Serving Size	Net Carb per Serving	GL per Serving
Pancakes, buckwheat, gluten-free, made from mix	102	2 4" pancakes	22	22
Pancakes, made from mix	67	2 4" pancakes	58	39
Papaya, fresh	59	4 oz	8	5
Parsnips	97	½ cup	12	12
Pastry	59	2 oz	26	15
Pea soup, canned	66	8 oz	41	27
Peach, canned in heavy syrup	58	½ cup	26	15
Peach, canned in light syrup	52	½ cup	18	9
Peach, fresh, large	42	4 oz	11	5
Peanuts	14	1.75 oz	6	1
Pear halves, canned in natural juice	43	½ cup	13	5
Pear, fresh	38	4 oz	11	4
Peas, green, frozen, cooked	48	½ cup	7	3
Pecans	[0]	1.75 oz	0	0
Pepper, fresh, green or red	[0]	3 oz	0	0
Pineapple, fresh	66	4 oz	10	6
Pineapple juice, unsweetened	46	8 oz	34	15
Pinto beans, canned	45	⅔ cup	22	10
Pinto beans, dried, cooked	39	¾ cup	26	10
Pita bread, white	57	1 oz	17	10
Pizza, cheese	60	1 slice	27	16
Pizza, Super Supreme, pan (11.4% fat)	36	1 slice	24	9
Pizza, Super Supreme, thin and crispy (13.2% fat)	30	1 slice	22	7
Plums, fresh	39	2 medium	12	5
Pop Tarts™, double chocolate	70	1.8 oz pastry	36	25

[0] indicates that the food has so little carbohydrate that the GI value cannot be tested. The GL, therefore, is 0.

FOOD	GI Value	Nominal Serving Size	Net Carb per Serving	GL per Serving
Popcorn, plain, cooked in microwave oven	72	1½ cups	11	8
Pork	[0]	4 oz	0	0
Potato chips, plain, salted	54	2 oz	21	11
Potato, baked	85	5 oz	30	26
Potato, microwaved	82	5 oz	33	27
Pound cake (Sara Lee)	54	2 oz	28	15
PowerBar® (chocolate)	57	2.3 oz	42	24
Premium soda crackers	74	5 crackers	17	12
Pretzels	83	1 oz	20	16
Prunes, pitted	29	6	33	10
Pudding, instant, chocolate, made with whole milk	47	½ cup	24	11
Pudding, instant, vanilla, made with whole milk	40	½ cup	24	10
Puffed crispbread	81	1 oz	19	15
Puffed rice cakes, white	82	3 cakes	21	17
Puffed Wheat, breakfast cereal	80	2 cups	21	17
Pumpernickel rye kernel bread	41	1 oz	12	5
Pumpkin	75	3 oz	4	3

R

FOOD	GI Value	Nominal Serving Size	Net Carb per Serving	GL per Serving
Raisin Bran™, breakfast cereal	61	½ cup	19	12
Raisins	64	½ cup	44	28
Ravioli, meat-filled, cooked	39	6.5 oz	38	15
Red wine	[0]	3.5 oz	0	0
Red-skinned potato, peeled and microwaved on high for 6–7.5 min	79	5 oz	18	14
Red-skinned potato, peeled, boiled 35 min	88	5 oz	18	16
Red-skinned potato, peeled, mashed	91	5 oz	20	18

[0] indicates that the food has so little carbohydrate that the GI value cannot be tested. The GL, therefore, is 0.

FOOD	GI Value	Nominal Serving Size	Net Carb per Serving	GL per Serving
Resource Diabetic™, nutritional support product, vanilla (Novartis)	34	8 oz	23	8
Rice and corn pasta, gluten-free	76	1½ cups	49	37
Rice bran, extruded	19	1 oz	14	3
Rice cakes, white	78	3 cakes	21	17
Rice Krispies™, breakfast cereal	82	1¼ cups	26	22
Rice Krispies Treat™ bar	63	1 oz	24	15
Rice noodles, fresh, cooked	40	1½ cups	39	15
Rice, parboiled	72	1 cup	36	26
Rice pasta, brown, cooked 16 min	92	1½ cups	38	35
Rice vermicelli	58	1½ cups	39	22
Rolled oats	42	1 cup	21	9
Roll-Ups®, processed fruit snack	99	1 oz	25	24
Roman (cranberry) beans, fresh, cooked	46	¾ cup	18	8
Russet, baked potato	85	5 oz	30	26
Rutabaga, fresh, cooked	72	5 oz	10	7
Rye bread	58	1 oz	14	8
Ryvita® crackers	69	3 crackers	16	11

S

FOOD	GI Value	Nominal Serving Size	Net Carb per Serving	GL per Serving
Salami	[0]	4 oz	0	0
Salmon	[0]	4 oz	0	0
Sausages, fried	28	3.5 oz	3	1
Scones, plain	92	1 oz	9	8
Sebago potato, peeled, cooked	87	5 oz	17	14
Seeded rye bread	55	1 oz	13	7
Semolina, cooked (dry)	55	⅓ cup	50	28
Shellfish (shrimp, crab, lobster, etc.)	[0]	4 oz	0	0
Sherry	[0]	2 oz	0	0
Shortbread cookies	64	1 oz	16	10

[0] indicates that the food has so little carbohydrate that the GI value cannot be tested. The GL, therefore, is 0.

POCKET GUIDE TO CHILDHOOD DIABETES

FOOD	GI Value	Nominal Serving Size	Net Carb per Serving	GL per Serving
Shredded Wheat™, breakfast cereal	75	⅔ cup	20	15
Shredded Wheat™ biscuits	62	1 oz	18	11
Skim milk	32	8 oz	13	4
Skittles®	70	45 pcs	45	32
Smacks™, breakfast cereal	71	¾ cup	23	11
Smoothie, raspberry (ConAgra)	33	8 oz	41	14
Snack bar, Apple Cinnamon (ConAgra)	40	1.75 oz	29	12
Snack bar, Peanut Butter & Choc-Chip (ConAgra)	37	1.75 oz	27	10
Snickers® bar	68	2.2 oz	35	23
Social Tea Biscuits	55	6 cookies	19	10
Soda crackers, Premium	74	5 crackers	17	12
Soft drink, Coca Cola®	53	8 oz	26	14
Soft drink, Fanta®, orange	68	8 oz	34	23
Sourdough rye	48	1 oz	12	6
Sourdough wheat	54	1 oz	14	8
Soy & Flaxseed bread (mix in bread oven) (ConAgra)	50	1 oz	10	5
Soybeans, canned	14	1 cup	6	1
Soybeans, dried, cooked	20	1 cup	6	1
Spaghetti, durum wheat, cooked 20 min	64	1½ cups	43	27
Spaghetti, gluten-free, rice and split pea, canned in tomato sauce	68	8 oz	27	19
Spaghetti, white, cooked 5 min	38	1½ cups	48	18
Spaghetti, whole wheat, cooked 5 min	32	1½ cups	44	14
Special K™, breakfast cereal	69	1 cup	21	14
Spirali pasta, durum wheat, al dente	43	1½ cups	44	19
Split pea and soy pasta shells, gluten-free	29	1½ cups	31	9
Split pea soup	60	1 cup	27	16

[0] indicates that the food has so little carbohydrate that the GI value cannot be tested. The GL, therefore, is 0.

FOOD	GI Value	Nominal Serving Size	Net Carb per Serving	GL per Serving
Split peas, yellow, cooked 20 min	32	¾ cup	19	6
Sponge cake, plain	46	2 oz	36	17
Squash, raw	[0]	⅔ cup	0	0
Star pastina, white, cooked 5 min	38	1½ cups	48	18
Stay Trim™, whole-grain bread (Natural Ovens)	70	1 oz	15	10
100% Stone-ground whole-wheat bread	53	1 slice	13	7
Stoned Wheat Thins	67	14 crackers	17	12
Strawberries, fresh	40	4 oz	3	1
Strawberry jam	51	1½ Tbsps	20	10
Strawberry shortcake	42	2.2 oz	40	17
Stuffing, bread	74	1 oz	21	16
Sucrose	68	1 Tbsp	10	7
Super Supreme pizza, pan (11.4% fat)	36	1 slice	24	9
Super Supreme pizza, thin and crispy (13.2% fat)	30	1 slice	22	7
Sushi, salmon	48	3.5 oz	36	17
Sweet corn, whole kernel, canned, diet-pack, drained	46	1 cup	28	13
Sweet potato, cooked	44	5 oz	25	11

T

FOOD	GI Value	Nominal Serving Size	Net Carb per Serving	GL per Serving
Taco shells, baked	68	2 shells	12	8
Tapioca, cooked with milk	81	¾ cup	18	14
Tofu-based frozen dessert, chocolate with high-fructose (24%) corn syrup	115	1.75 oz	9	10
Tomato juice, canned, no added sugar	38	8 oz	9	4
Tomato soup	38	1 cup	17	6
Tortellini, cheese	50	6.5 oz	21	10
Tortilla chips, plain, salted	63	1.75 oz	26	17
Total™, breakfast cereal	76	¾ cup	22	17
Tuna	[0]	4 oz	0	0

[0] indicates that the food has so little carbohydrate that the GI value cannot be tested. The GL, therefore, is 0.

POCKET GUIDE TO CHILDHOOD DIABETES

FOOD	GI Value	Nominal Serving Size	Net Carb per Serving	GL per Serving
Twix® Cookie Bar, caramel	44	2 cookies	39	17
U				
Ultra chocolate ice cream, premium, 15% fat	37	½ cup	14	5
Ultracal™ with fiber (Mead Johnson)	40	8 oz	29	12
V				
Vanilla cake made from mix, with vanilla frosting	42	4 oz	58	24
Vanilla pudding, instant, made with whole milk	40	½ cup	24	10
Vanilla wafers, creme-filled, FIFTY50	41	4 cookies	20	8
Vanilla wafers	77	6 cookies	18	14
Veal	[0]	4 oz	0	0
Vermicelli, white, cooked	35	1½ cups	44	16
W				
Waffles, Aunt Jemima®	76	1 4" waffle	13	10
Walnuts	[0]	1.75 oz	0	0
Water crackers	78	7 crackers	18	14
Watermelon, fresh	72	4 oz	6	4
Weet-Bix™, breakfast cereal	69	2 biscuits	17	12
Wheaties™, breakfast cereal	82	1 cup	21	17
Whiskey	[0]	1 oz	0	0
White bread	70	1 oz	14	10
White rice, instant, cooked 6 min	87	1 cup	42	36
White wine	[0]	3.5 oz	0	0
100% Whole Grain™ bread (Natural Ovens)	51	1 oz	13	7
Whole milk	31	8 oz	12	4
Whole-wheat bread	77	1 oz	12	9
Wonder™ white bread	80	1 oz	14	11

[0] indicates that the food has so little carbohydrate that the GI value cannot be tested. The GL, therefore, is 0.

FOOD	GI Value	Nominal Serving Size	Net Carb per Serving	GL per Serving
X				
Xylitol	8	1 Tbsp	10	1
Y				
Yam, peeled, cooked	37	5 oz	36	13
Yogurt, low-fat, wild strawberry	31	8 oz	34	11
Yogurt, low-fat, with fruit and artificial sweetener	14	8 oz	15	2
Yogurt, low-fat, with fruit and sugar	33	8 oz	35	12

[0] indicates that the food has so little carbohydrate that the GI value cannot be tested. The GL, therefore, is 0.

38

YOUR LOW-GI FOOD FINDER

A high GI value is 70 or more.
An intermediate GI value is 56 to 69 inclusive.
A low GI value is 55 or less.

	11–20	21–30	31–40	41–50	51–55
	11–20				
Peanut Butter	14				
Peanuts	14				
Soybeans	14				
Yogurt	14				
Fructose	19				
Maple Syrup	19				
Rice Bran	19				

GI VALUE 11–20 21–30 31–40 41–50 51–55

21–30

Food	GI
Cashews	22
Cherries	22
Choice DM™ Beverage, Mead Johnson	23
Kidney Beans	23
Barley	25
Grapefruit	25
Lentils	26
Apples, Dried	29
Prunes, Dried	29
Black Beans	30
Hearty Oatmeal Cookies	30

31–40

Food	GI
Apricots, Dried	31
Butter Beans	31
Chocolate, Milk, Sugar-Free, Fifty50	31
Soy Milk	31
Lima Beans	32
Milk, Skim	32
Spaghetti, Whole Wheat	32
Split Peas, Dried	32
M&M's™ Peanut	33
Nutella®	33
Milk, Low-fat Chocolate	34
Hearty Chocolate Meal Replacement Drink	35
Ice Cream, Low-fat	37
Yam	37
All-Bran®	38

POCKET GUIDE TO CHILDHOOD DIABETES

GI VALUE

	11–20	21–30	31–40	41–50	51–55
Cannellini Beans			38		
Navy Beans			38		
Pastina			38		
Peaches, Canned			38		
Pears			38		
Rice, Converted			38		
Tomato Juice			38		
Tomato Soup			38		
Mung Beans			39		
Plums			39		
Ravioli			39		
Apple Juice			40		
Apples			40		
Fettuccine, Egg			40		
Strawberries			40		

	41–50
Bread, Pumpernickel	41
Crème Filled Wafers, Vanilla	41
Black-eyed Peas	42
Chickpeas	42
Peaches	42
Spaghetti, Durum Wheat	42
Chocolate, Milk	43
Custard	43
Pudding	43
Lentil Soup	44
Capellini	45
Pinto Beans	45
Corn	46

	11–20	21–30	31–40	41–50	51–55
Grapes				46	
Lactose				46	
Sponge Cake				46	
All-Bran Bran Buds				47	
Macaroni				47	
Baked Beans				48	
Bulgur				48	
Grapefruit Juice				48	
Orange Marmalade				48	
Oranges				48	
Peas, Green				48	
Sweet Potato				48	
Pears, Canned				49	
Muesli				49	
Oat Bran Breakfast Cereal				50	
Rice, Brown				50	
Tortellini, Cheese, Frozen				50	

	51–55
All Bran with Extra Fiber	51
Bread, 100% Whole Grain	51
Mangoes	51
Oatmeal, Old-Fashioned	51
Strawberry Jam	51
Kidney Beans, Canned	52
Linguine, Thick	52
Spaghetti with Meat Sauce	52
Sushi	52
Bread, Sourdough Rye	53
Bread, Stone-ground 100% Whole-Wheat	53
Kiwi, Fresh	53

GI VALUE — 11–20, 21–30, 31–40, 41–50, 51–55

Food	GI
Bread, Sourdough Wheat	54
Buckwheat	54
Oatmeal Cookies	54
Pound Cake	54
Rice, Long Grain and Wild	54
Fruit Cocktail	55
Honey	55
Oat Bran, Raw	55
Semolina	55
Social Tea Biscuits	55

◀ 39 ▶

LOW- TO HIGH-GI VALUES

For those who wish to choose a diet with the lowest GI values possible, we've created the following listing in order of GI values (i.e., from lowest to highest value). We've also divided the list into food categories, so that when you want to find a low-GI vegetable or fruit, for example, the information is at your fingertips. The categories are:

- bakery products
- beverages
- breads
- breakfast foods
- cookies
- crackers
- dairy products and alternatives
- fruits and fruit products
- grains
- infant formulas and baby foods

- legumes
- meal-replacement products
- mixed meals and convenience foods
- noodles
- pasta
- protein foods
- snack foods and candy
- soups
- special dietary products
- sugars
- vegetables

As we discuss in *The New Glucose Revolution,* it's not necessary to eat all of your carbohydrates from low-GI sources. If half of your carbohydrate choices have low-GI values, you're doing well. If you also eat a low-GI food at each meal, you'll be reducing the GI values overall.

FOOD	LOW	INTERMEDIATE	HIGH

BAKERY PRODUCTS

Cakes

Food	Low	Intermediate	High
Banana	○		
Chocolate, with chocolate frosting	○		
Pound	○		
Sponge	○		
Vanilla	○		
Angel food		◐	
Flan		◐	

Muffins

Food	Low	Intermediate	High
Apple, with sugar or artificial sweeteners	○		
Apple, oat, and raisin	○		
Banana, oat, and honey		◐	
Bran		◐	
Blueberry		◐	
Carrot		◐	
Oatmeal, made from mix, Quaker Oats		◐	
Cupcake, iced			●
Scone, plain			●

Pastries

Food	Low	Intermediate	High
Croissant		◐	
Doughnut, cake-type			●

BEVERAGES

Alcoholic

Food	Low	Intermediate	High
Beer	○		
Brandy	○		

FOOD	LOW	INTERMEDIATE	HIGH
Gin	○		
Sherry	○		
Whiskey	○		
Wine, red	○		
Wine, white	○		

Juices

Apple, with sugar or artificial sweetener	○		
Carrot, fresh	○		
Grapefruit, unsweetened	○		
Pineapple, unsweetened	○		
Tomato, canned, no added sugar	○		

Smoothies and shakes

Raspberry	○		
Soy	○		

Soft drinks

Coca-Cola®		◐	
Fanta®		◐	

Sports drinks

Gatorade®			●

BREADS

Fruit

Muesli, made from mix	○		
Happiness™, cinnamon, raisin, pecan		◐	

Gluten-free

Fiber-enriched			●
White			●

FOOD	LOW	INTERMEDIATE	HIGH
Rye			
Pumpernickel	○		
Sourdough	○		
Cocktail		◐	
Light		◐	
Whole-wheat		◐	
Spelt			
Multigrain	○		
White			●
Wheat			
100% Stone-ground whole-wheat bread	○		
100% Whole Grain	○		
Soy & Linseed bread machine mix	○		
Flatbread, Indian		◐	
Hearty 7 Grain		◐	
Pita, plain		◐	
Bagel			●
Baguette			●
Bread stuffing			●
English muffin			●
Flatbread, Middle Eastern			●
Italian			●
Lebanese, white			●
White, enriched			●
Whole-wheat			●

POCKET GUIDE TO CHILDHOOD DIABETES

FOOD	LOW	INTERMEDIATE	HIGH
BREAKFAST FOODS			
Breakfast cereal bars			
Rice Krispies® Treat		◐	
Cooked cereals			
Hot cereal, apple & cinnamon, ConAgra	○		
Old-fashioned oats	○		
Cream of Wheat™, regular, Nabisco		◐	
One Minute Oats, Quaker Oats		◐	
Quick Oats, Quaker Oats		◐	
Cream of Wheat™, instant, Nabisco			●
Oatmeal, instant			●
Grain products			
Pancakes, prepared from mix	○		
Pancakes, buckwheat, gluten-free, made from mix			●
Waffles, Aunt Jemima®			●
Ready-to-eat cereals			
All-Bran®, Kellogg's	○		
Complete™ Bran Flakes, Kellogg's	○		
Bran Buds™, Kellogg's		◐	
Bran Chex™, Kellogg's		◐	
Froot Loops™, Kellogg's		◐	
Frosted Flakes™, Kellogg's		◐	
Just Right™, Kellogg's		◐	
Life™, Quaker Oats		◐	
Nutrigrain™, Kellogg's		◐	
Oat bran, raw, Quaker Oats		◐	
Puffed Wheat, Quaker Oats		◐	

FOOD	LOW	INTERMEDIATE	HIGH
Raisin Bran™, Kellogg's		◐	
Special K™, Kellogg's		◐	
Bran Flakes™, Kellogg's			●
Cheerios™, General Mills			●
Corn Chex™, Kellogg's			●
Corn Flakes™, Kellogg's			●
Corn Pops™, Kellogg's			●
Grapenuts™, Post			●
Rice Krispies™, Kellogg's			●
Shredded Wheat™, Nabisco			●
Team™ Flakes, Nabisco			●
Total™			●
Weetabix™			●

COOKIES

FOOD	LOW	INTERMEDIATE	HIGH
Hearty Oatmeal, F<small>IFTY</small>50	○		
Oatmeal, Sugar-Free, F<small>IFTY</small>50	○		
Social Tea Biscuits	○		
Vanilla wafers, creme filled, F<small>IFTY</small>50	○		
Arrowroot		◐	
Digestives		◐	
Shortbread		◐	
Vanilla wafers			●

CRACKERS

FOOD	LOW	INTERMEDIATE	HIGH
Breton wheat		◐	
Melba toast		◐	
Rye crispbread		◐	
Ryvita™		◐	
Stoned Wheat Thins		◐	
Water		◐	

FOOD	LOW	INTERMEDIATE	HIGH
Kavli™ Norwegian Crispbread			●
Premium soda (Saltines)			●
Rice cakes, puffed			●

DAIRY PRODUCTS AND ALTERNATIVES

Custard

Homemade	○		

Ice cream

Regular	○		

Milk

Low-fat, chocolate, with aspartame	○		
Low-fat, chocolate, with sugar	○		
Skim	○		
Whole	○		
Condensed, sweetened			●

Mousse

Butterscotch, low-fat, Nestlé	○		
Chocolate, low-fat, Nestlé	○		
French vanilla, low-fat, Nestlé	○		
Hazelnut, low-fat, Nestlé	○		
Mango, low-fat, Nestlé	○		
Mixed berry, low-fat, Nestlé	○		
Strawberry, low-fat, Nestlé	○		

Pudding

Instant, chocolate, made with milk	○		
Instant, vanilla, made with milk	○		

FOOD	LOW	INTERMEDIATE	HIGH
Soy milk			
Reduced-fat	○		
Whole	○		
Soy yogurt			
Tofu-based frozen dessert, chocolate			●
Yogurt			
Low-fat, fruit, with aspartame	○		
Low-fat, fruit, with sugar	○		
Nonfat, French vanilla, with sugar	○		
Nonfat, strawberry, with sugar	○		

FRUIT AND FRUIT PRODUCTS

FOOD	LOW	INTERMEDIATE	HIGH
Apple, fresh	○		
Apricot, fresh	○		
Banana, fresh	○		
Cantaloupe, fresh	○		
Cherries, fresh	○		
Grapefruit, fresh	○		
Grapes, fresh	○		
Kiwi, fresh	○		
Mango, fresh	○		
Orange, fresh	○		
Peach, canned in natural juice	○		
Peach, fresh	○		
Pear, canned in pear juice	○		
Pear, fresh	○		
Plum, fresh	○		
Prunes, pitted	○		
Strawberries, fresh	○		
Strawberry jam	○		
Figs, dried		◐	

POCKET GUIDE TO CHILDHOOD DIABETES

FOOD	LOW	INTERMEDIATE	HIGH
Fruit cocktail, canned		◑	
Papaya, fresh		◑	
Peach, canned in heavy syrup		◑	
Peach, canned in light syrup		◑	
Pineapple, fresh		◑	
Raisins/sultanas		◑	
Dates, dried			●
Lychee, canned in syrup, drained			●
Watermelon, fresh			●

GRAINS

FOOD	LOW	INTERMEDIATE	HIGH
Barley, cracked	○		
Barley, pearled	○		
Buckwheat	○		
Buckwheat groats	○		
Bulgur	○		
Corn, canned, no salt added	○		
Rice, brown	○		
Rice, Cajun Style, Uncle Ben's®	○		
Rice, Long Grain and Wild, Uncle Ben's®	○		
Rice, parboiled, converted, white, cooked 20–30 min, Uncle Ben's®	○		
Barley, rolled		◑	
Corn, fresh		◑	
Cornmeal		◑	
Couscous		◑	
Rice, arborio (risotto)		◑	
Rice, Basmati		◑	
Rice, Garden Style, Uncle Ben's®		◑	
Rice, parboiled, long-grain, cooked 10 minutes		◑	
Millet			●

FOOD	LOW	INTERMEDIATE	HIGH
Rice, sticky			●
Rice, parboiled			●
Tapioca, boiled with milk			●

INFANT FORMULA AND BABY FOODS

Baby foods

	LOW	INTERMEDIATE	HIGH
Apple, apricot, and banana, baby cereal		◐	
Chicken and noodles with vegetables, strained		◐	
Corn and rice, baby		◐	
Oatmeal, creamed, baby		◐	
Rice pudding, baby		◐	

Infant formula

	LOW	INTERMEDIATE	HIGH
SMA, 20 cal./fl oz, Wyeth	○		
Nursoy, soy-based, milk-free, Wyeth		◐	

LEGUMES

Beans

	LOW	INTERMEDIATE	HIGH
Baked, canned	○		
Butter, dried and cooked	○		
Kidney, canned	○		
Lima, baby, frozen	○		
Mung, cooked	○		
Navy, dried and cooked	○		
Pinto, cooked	○		
Soy, canned	○		

Lentils

	LOW	INTERMEDIATE	HIGH
Green, dried and cooked	○		
Red, dried and cooked	○		

POCKET GUIDE TO CHILDHOOD DIABETES

FOOD	LOW	INTERMEDIATE	HIGH

Peas

Black-eyed	○		
Chickpeas/garbanzo beans, canned	○		
Split, yellow, cooked	○		

MEAL-REPLACEMENT PRODUCTS

Designer chocolate, sugar-free, Worldwide Sport Nutrition low-carbohydrate products	○		
L.E.A.N Fibergy™ bar, Harvest Oat, Usana	○		
L.E.A.N (Life long) Nutribar™, Peanut Crunch, Usana	○		
L.E.A.N (Life long) Nutribar™, Chocolate Crunch, Usana	○		

MIXED MEALS AND CONVENIENCE FOODS

Chicken nuggets, frozen, reheated	○		
Fish fillet, reduced fat, breaded	○		
Fish sticks	○		
Greek lentil stew with a bread roll, homemade	○		
Lean Cuisine™, chicken with rice	○		
Pizza, Super Supreme, pan, Pizza Hut	○		
Pizza, Super Supreme, thin and crispy, Pizza Hut	○		
Pizza, Vegetarian Supreme, thin and crispy, Pizza Hut	○		
Spaghetti Bolognese	○		
Sushi, salmon	○		
Tortellini, cheese, Stouffer	○		
Tuna patty, reduced fat	○		
Cheese sandwich, white bread		◐	
Kugel		◐	
Macaroni and cheese, boxed, Kraft		◐	
Peanut-butter sandwich, white/whole-wheat bread		◐	
Pizza, cheese, Pillsbury		◐	

163

THE NEW GLUCOSE REVOLUTION

FOOD	LOW	INTERMEDIATE	HIGH
Spaghetti, gluten-free, canned in tomato sauce		◐	
Sushi, roasted sea algae, vinegar and rice		◐	
Taco shells, cornmeal-based, baked, El Paso		◐	
White bread and butter		◐	
Stir-fried vegetables with chicken and rice, homemade			●

NOODLES

FOOD	LOW	INTERMEDIATE	HIGH
Instant	○		
Mung bean, Lungkow beanthread	○		
Rice, fresh, cooked	○		
Rice, dried, cooked		◐	
Udon, plain, reheated 5 min		◐	

PASTA

FOOD	LOW	INTERMEDIATE	HIGH
Capellini	○		
Fettuccine, egg	○		
Gluten-free, cornstarch	○		
Linguine, thick, fresh, durum wheat, white	○		
Linguine, thin, fresh, durum wheat	○		
Macaroni, plain, cooked	○		
Ravioli	○		
Spaghetti, cooked 5 min	○		
Spaghetti, cooked 22 min	○		
Spaghetti, protein-enriched, cooked 7 min	○		
Spaghetti, whole-wheat	○		
Spirali, cooked, durum wheat	○		
Star pastina, cooked 5 min	○		
Tortellini	○		
Vermicelli	○		
Gnocchi		◐	

POCKET GUIDE TO CHILDHOOD DIABETES

FOOD	LOW	INTERMEDIATE	HIGH
Rice vermicelli		◐	
Spaghetti, cooked 10 min, Barilla		◐	
Corn, gluten-free			●
Rice and corn, gluten-free			●
Rice, brown, cooked 16 min			●

PROTEIN FOODS

FOOD	LOW	INTERMEDIATE	HIGH
Beef	○		
Cheese	○		
Cold cuts	○		
Eggs	○		
Fish	○		
Lamb	○		
Pork	○		
Sausages	○		
Shellfish (shrimp, crab, lobster, etc.)	○		
Veal	○		

SNACK FOODS AND CANDY

Candy

FOOD	LOW	INTERMEDIATE	HIGH
Nougat	○		
Jelly beans			●
Life Savers®			●
Skittles®			●

Chips

FOOD	LOW	INTERMEDIATE	HIGH
Corn, plain, salted, Doritos™	○		
Potato, plain, salted	○		

Chocolate bars

FOOD	LOW	INTERMEDIATE	HIGH
Milk, Cadbury's	○		

FOOD	LOW	INTERMEDIATE	HIGH
Milk, Dove®, Mars	○		
Milk, Nestlé	○		
White, Milky Bar®	○		
Mars Bar®			◐
Snickers Bar®			◐

Chocolate candy

M & M's®, peanut	○		

Chocolate spread

Nutella®, chocolate hazelnut spread	○		

Dried-fruit bars

Fruit Roll-Ups®			●

Nuts

Cashews	○		
Peanuts	○		
Pecans	○		

Popcorn

Plain, microwaved			●

Pretzels

Plain, salted			●

Snack bars

Apple Cinnamon, ConAgra	○		
Peanut Butter & Choc-Chip	○		
Twix® Cookie Bar, caramel	○		
Kudos Whole Grain Bars, chocolate chip		◐	

Sports bars

Ironman PR bar®, chocolate	○		

POCKET GUIDE TO CHILDHOOD DIABETES

FOOD	LOW	INTERMEDIATE	HIGH
PowerBar®, chocolate		◐	

SOUPS

FOOD	LOW	INTERMEDIATE	HIGH
Lentil, canned	○		
Minestrone, canned, ready-to-serve	○		
Tomato, canned	○		
Black bean, canned		◐	
Green pea, canned		◐	
Split pea, canned		◐	

SPECIAL DIETARY PRODUCTS

FOOD	LOW	INTERMEDIATE	HIGH
Choice DM™, vanilla, Mead Johnson	○		
Ensure™, Abbott	○		
Ensure Plus™, vanilla, Abbott	○		
Ensure Pudding™, vanilla, Abbott	○		
Ensure™ bar, chocolate fudge brownie, Abbott	○		
Ensure™, vanilla, Abbott	○		
Glucerna™ bar, lemon crunch, Abbott	○		
Glucerna™ SR shake, vanilla, Abbott	○		
Glucerna™, vanilla, Abbott	○		
Resource Diabetic™, vanilla, Novartis	○		
Resource Plus, chocolate, Novartis	○		
Ultracal™ with fiber, Mead Johnson	○		
Enercal Plus™, Wyeth-Ayerst		◐	
Enrich Plus shake, vanilla, Ross		◐	

SUGARS

FOOD	LOW	INTERMEDIATE	HIGH
Blue Agave, Organic Agave Cactus Nectar, light, 90% fructose, Western Commerce	○		
Blue Agave, Organic Agave Cactus Nectar, light, 97% fructose, Western Commerce	○		
Fructose	○		

THE NEW GLUCOSE REVOLUTION

FOOD	LOW	INTERMEDIATE	HIGH
Lactose	○		
Honey		◐	
Sucrose		◐	
Glucose			●
Maltose			●

VEGETABLES

FOOD	LOW	INTERMEDIATE	HIGH
Artichokes	○		
Avocado	○		
Bok choy	○		
Broccoli	○		
Cabbage	○		
Carrots, peeled, cooked	○		
Cassava (yucca), cooked with salt	○		
Cauliflower	○		
Celery	○		
Corn, canned, no salt added	○		
Cucumber	○		
French beans (runner beans)	○		
Leafy greens	○		
Lettuce	○		
Peas, frozen, cooked	○		
Pepper	○		
Potato, sweet	○		
Squash	○		
Yam	○		
Beet		◐	
Corn, sweet, cooked		◐	
Potato, boiled/canned		◐	
Potato, new, canned		◐	
Taro		◐	

FOOD	LOW	INTERMEDIATE	HIGH
Broad beans			●
Parsnips			●
Potato, French fries, frozen and reheated			●
Potato, instant			●
Potato, mashed			●
Potato, microwaved			●
Potato, russet, baked			●
Pumpkin			●
Rutabaga			●

FOR MORE INFORMATION

To find a dietitian
The American Dietetic Association
120 S. Riverside Plaza
Suite 2000
Chicago, IL 60606
Phone: 1-800-877-1600
www.eatright.org

To order Natural Ovens bread
Natural Ovens Bakery
PO Box 730
Manitowoc, WI 54221-0730
Phone: 1-800-772-0730
www.naturalovens.com

To order Fifty50 Foods or find your nearest retailer
Fifty50 Foods

PO Box 89
Mendham, NJ 07945
Phone: 1-973-543-7006
www.fifty50.com

Primary Care Physicians

If you think you need help with a weight problem, it's always a good idea to see your primary care physician for an evaluation.

Community Support Groups

Many communities offer support groups targeting people who are trying to lose weight. Your primary care physician or local hospital may be able to direct you to a support group best suited to your needs.

Diabetes Organizations

Extra weight can often make a diabetic condition worse. For more information about living with and controlling your diabetes, contact the following:

The American Diabetes Association
1701 North Beauregard Street
Alexandria, VA 22311
Phone: 1-800-DIABETES (1-800-342-2383)
http://www.diabetes.org/

Canadian Diabetes Association
National Office
15 Toronto Street, Suite 800
Toronto, ON M5C 2E3
Phone: 1-416-363-3373
1-800-BANTING (1-800-226-8464)
http://www.diabetes.ca/

GLYCEMIC INDEX TESTING

*I*F YOU ARE a food manufacturer, you may be interested in having the glycemic index value of some of your products tested on a fee-for-service basis. For more information, contact:

Sydney University Glycaemic Index Research Service (SUGiRS)
Department of Biochemistry
University of Sydney
NSW 2006 Australia
Fax: (61) (2) 9351-6022
E-mail: j.brandmiller@mmb.usyd.edu.au

ABOUT THE AUTHORS

JENNIE BRAND-MILLER, PH.D., is Professor of Human Nutrition in the Human Nutrition Unit, School of Molecular and Microbial Biosciences at the University of Sydney, and President of the Nutrition Society of Australia. She has taught postgraduate students of nutrition and dietetics at the University of Sydney for over twenty-four years and currently leads a team of twelve research scientists, whose interests focus on all aspects of carbohydrate—diet and diabetes, the glycemic index of foods, insulin resistance, lactose intolerance, and oligosaccharides in infant nutrition. She has published sixteen books and 140 journal articles and is the co-author of all books in the Glucose Revolution series.

■

KAYE FOSTER-POWELL, M. NUTR. & DIET., is an accredited practicing dietitian with extensive experience in diabetes management. She has conducted research into the glycemic index of foods and its practical applications over the last fifteen years. Currently she is a dietitian with Wentworth Area Diabetes Services in New South Wales and consults on all aspects of the glycemic index. She is the co-author of all books in the Glucose Revolution series.

■

Heather Gilbertson, B. Sc., Grad. Dip. Diet., Grad. Cert. Ed., APD, is a clinical specialist dietitian and diabetes dietitian educator with over 12 years of clinical experience in diabetes management in children and adolescents at the Royal Children's Hospital Women's and Children's Health Care Network, Melbourne. Her Ph.D. research evaluated the effect of low GI and measured carbohydrate diets in children with diabetes. She also conducts a private practice in the Macedon Ranges, Victoria.

ACKNOWLEDGMENTS

We would like to thank Linda Rao, M.Ed., for her editorial work on the American edition.

Also Available

More than 2 MILLION Glucose Revolution Titles Sold Worldwide!

THE NEW GLUCOSE REVOLUTION

The Authoritative Guide to the Glycemic Index—the Dietary Solution for Lifelong Health

ISBN 1-56924-506-1 • $15.95

Written by the world's leading authorities on the subject, whose findings are supported by hundreds of studies from Harvard University's School of Public Health and other leading research centers, *The New Glucose Revolution* shows how and why eating low-GI foods has major health benefits for everybody seeking to establish a way of eating for lifelong health.

New York Times bestseller

THE GLUCOSE REVOLUTION LIFE PLAN

Discover how to make the glycemic index —the most significant dietary finding of the last 25 years— the foundation for a lifetime of healthy eating

More than 80,000 copies sold!

ISBN 1-56924-609-2 • $18.95

Both an introduction to the benefits of low-GI foods and an essential source for those already familiar with the concept, *The Glucose Revolution Life Plan* presents the glycemic index within the context of today's full nutrition picture.